GW00669511

THE WORLD TRAVELLERS'
MANUAL OF HOMOEOPATHY

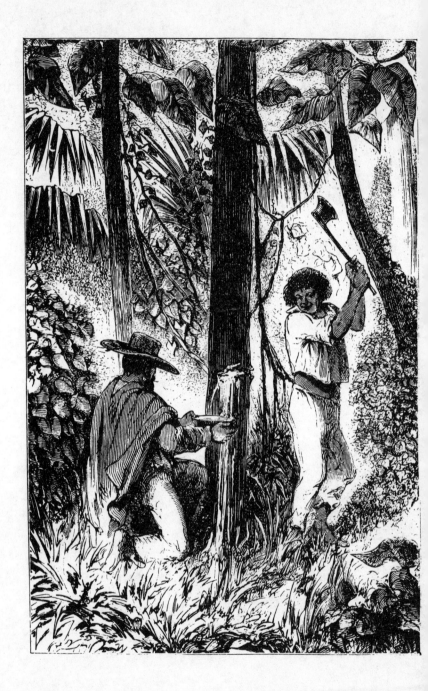

THE WORLD TRAVELLERS' MANUAL OF HOMOEOPATHY

Dr Colin B. Lessell
MB, BS(Lond), BDS(Lond), MRCS(Eng),
LRCP(Lond)

INDEX COMPILED BY
LYN GREENWOOD

SAFFRON WALDEN
THE C.W. DANIEL COMPANY LIMITED

Other books by the same author

Homoeopathy for Physicians
The Dental Prescriber
Die homöopathische Verordnung in der zahnärtzlichen Praxis
The Biochemic Handbook
Handbuch der homöopathischen Gewebesalze
The Traveller's Prescriber

To
those members of my family
who supported me in the preparation
of this manual

First published in Great Britain in 1993
by The C. W. Daniel Company Limited
1 Church Path, Saffron Walden
Essex, CB10 1JP, England

© Colin B. Lessell 1993

ISBN 0 85207 242 2

The illustrations in the text are from
On the Banks of the Amazon
by W. H. G. Kingston
published in 1873 by
T. Nelson & Sons, Paternoster Row, London
By courtesy of Herr Heinz Storch

Frontis: Extracting milk from a cow-tree

This book is printed on part-recycled paper

Designed by Tim McPhee
Produced by Book Production Consultants, Cambridge.
Typeset in Times by Rowland Phototypesetting Limited,
Bury St Edmunds, Suffolk and printed by
St Edmundsbury Press Limited, Bury St Edmunds, Suffolk.
The cover was printed on PVC
by The White Crescent Press, Luton, Beds
who specialise in printing on synthetic materials.

CONTENTS

PREFACE

This manual has been written not only to serve the needs of the average traveller, but also those of the more adventurous, who may embark upon journeys to tropical, remote, or impoverished areas of the globe. Indeed, with an increasing taste for the exotic, the distinction between the average and the adventurous traveller is becoming less clear, and many ordinary citizens now expose themselves to an increasing number of health hazards, with which they should make themselves familiar.

To these ends are described the geographical distribution, modes of transmission, methods of prevention, and clinical pictures of a wide range of illnesses, together with considerable details of appropriate homoeopathic treatments, and other safe forms of therapy.

Whilst this manual is primarily intended for the traveller, its content should also be found valuable for the residents, physicians, nurses, missionaries, and paramedics of developing, isolated, or heavily-diseased areas, in those situations where orthodox treatments are unacceptable, unsatisfactory, unavailable, or unknown.

Furthermore, should any of my readers have any new or corroboratory observations with regard to the homoeopathic or botanic (herbal) treatment of exotic diseases, I would be pleased to receive them via the publishers (please address your comments to: Dr C. B. Lessell, c/o C. W. Daniel Co. Ltd, 1 Church Path, Saffron Walden, Essex CB10 1JP, England).

Indeed, it is true to say that this manual could not have been properly formulated without some valuable personal communications. My thanks must go to: Mr Tony Pinkus, Dr Evelyn Eglington, and Mrs Audrey Ulbricht of Ainsworths Pharmacy, London, England; Mr and Mrs Peter Janssen of Bedford, England; Mr and Mrs Warwick Williams, and Mr Digby Woods, formerly of central Africa; Mr Bill Davies, explorer; Dr Wiley Gibbs of Australia; and many others, especially those from remote areas, who replied to my enquiries. Mrs Mary Gooch of the Glasgow Homoeopathic Library is to be thanked for seeking and supplying relevant material. Most particularly, I am indebted to Dr David Lilley of South Africa for his unique communication on the homoeopathic treatment of bilharziasis, which I have quoted in the text with only minor modifications.

Dr C. B. Lessell,
MB, BS, BDS, MRCS, LRCP

INTRODUCTION

This manual is truly dedicated to the needs of the modern traveller. Whatever the mode of travel or destination, be it beach, mountain, or jungle, it will serve as an indispensable companion.

With regard to both the *common and exotic* diseases associated with travel, you will learn:

How to prevent disease.
How to identify disease.
Practical first-aid measures.
How to treat safely and effectively with homoeopathic and herbal remedies.

Concerning *treatment*, this manual will provide you with:

**The ability to treat non-serious disease.*
**The ability to provide emergency treatment for serious disease, whilst awaiting expert medical assistance.*
**The ability to treat serious disease where expert medical advice is unavailable.*
**Sufficient basic information on the prescription of natural remedies.*

You are strongly advised to seek expert medical assistance in the case of serious or potentially serious disease.

Please read sections 1 and 2 of this manual carefully, concerning the use of natural medicines, before attempting to prescribe.

Items in small print
These are generally of a special medical nature (such as points of differential diagnosis, or descriptions of relatively rare diseases), or contain information more relevant to those with homoeopathic experience, or homoeopathic pharmacists.

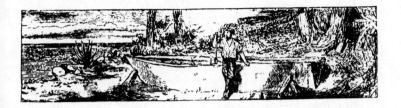

Section 1

BASIC HOMOEOPATHIC PRESCRIBING FOR TRAVELLERS

The majority of prescriptions given in this book concern the use of homoeopathic remedies.

Homoeopathic remedies are particularly suited to the needs of the global traveller in the following respects:

Basic prescribing is easy to learn.
Correctly prescribed, they are very safe.
They are suitable for young and old alike.
They are highly effective.
They are easy to administer.
They have a long shelf-life.
They are compact and light.
They are relatively easy to obtain, and are inexpensive.
They are legally transportable across international borders.
Their nomenclature is standardised world-wide.

A travelling wallet measuring 15cm × 10.5cm × 1.5cm, and

weighing a mere 200g, will contain 24 different remedies in 1g vials. Each 1g vial may contain up to 300 doses of the remedy.

Homoeopathic remedies are readily available without prescription in the United Kingdom, most other European countries, the USA, and India. Some difficulty may be found in obtaining certain remedies in Australia, New Zealand, and Italy. Whilst most general pharmacies and health-food stores now carry a reasonable range of homoeopathic remedies, the traveller may well need access to a specialised homoeopathic pharmacy, in order to obtain all requirements. Those listed at the end of this book offer an excellent postal service for both home and abroad. They will also prepare and supply general and individualised travel packs (see *Section 28* for a basic list of remedies).

Homoeopathic remedies are generally presented in the form of spherical pills (about 4mm in diameter), which are termed *pilules*, or flat *tablets*. These are administered by mouth, and have a pleasant taste. Other oral presentations include: *coarse granules, fine granules, powders, and liquids*.

Coarse granules (sometimes termed *globules*) are spherical and the size of a pin-head. A 1g vial contains approximately 300 coarse granules. Where compactness and lightness are a necessity, the traveller is advised to secure his remedies in this form. However, being so small, they are easily dropped and lost.

Pilules and tablets are more easily managed, but are a little more bulky. A standard 7g vial contains approximately 70 pilules.

Vials are composed of either plastic or glass. The shelf-life of a remedy tends to be better in glass than plastic, but glass is more likely to shatter. Whatever the relative virtues, most remedies are purchased in glass containers.

All remedies should be kept in their *original* vials, and stored away from *daylight* and highly aromatic substances. Provided the vials are tightly stoppered, subjection to heat presents no problem. Neither is severe cold problematical, except in the case of liquid preparations of low alcohol content, which may freeze, expand, and fracture their bottles. Remember, however, that the prolonged exposure of remedies to *sunlight* will render them ineffective. Correctly stored, their shelf-life is many years.

Homoeopathic remedies are largely derived from natural materials, most frequently vegetable or mineral. The methods of preparation of homoeopathic remedies preserve or enhance the medicinal properties of the original material, whilst reducing any toxicity to a negligible level. *Correctly administered*, they are completely safe for both children and adults.

The *nomenclature, or labelling*, of homoeopathic remedies requires some explanation, e.g:

"*Belladonna 30c*"

Belladonna is the latinized name of the original material, the plant *Deadly Nightshade*. With but a few exceptions, remedies are sold under their latinized names in all homoeopathic pharmacies throughout the World, thus minimizing the linguistic barriers to their purchase. The numerical expression *30c* is the *potency* of the remedy, or strength. The higher the numerical value, the greater the strength of medicinal action.

Homoeopathic remedies are prepared by a system which involves dilution. The letter *c*, which follows the number *30*, refers to the method of dilution by which the remedy was prepared. It stands for *centesimal scale*. By custom, the suffix *c* is often omitted. In French-speaking countries, the abbreviation *CH* is used to denote the centesimal scale. Hence,

$$30c = 30 = 30\ CH$$

Remedies may also be obtained which have been prepared on the *decimal scale* of dilution, denoted by the suffix *x*. Hence, we may purchase:

Belladonna 30x

In northern Europe, the suffix *x* is replaced by the prefix *D*. Thus,

$$30x = D30$$

For any given potency number, the *x* potency is slightly

weaker in medicinal action than the *c* potency. However, for most practical purposes, this therapeutic difference may be ignored. From the point of view of the traveller, we may make the approximation:

Belladonna 30c = Belladonna 30x

Some words of **caution** are now in order. When purchasing lower potencies of remedies that are made from essentially *toxic* materials, such as *Deadly Nightshade*, observe the following rule: **Do not obtain such remedies in potencies less than 12x (D12) on the decimal scale, or less than 6c (6, 6 CH) on the centesimal scale**. Numerical values equal to, or *greater* than those stated signify *negligible toxicity*.

The most commonly available and most commonly used potencies are *6c* and *30c*.

Occasionally, homoeopathic remedies are utilized in the form of *mother tincture*. This is the undiluted alcoholic extract of a material, usually a plant. The symbol for mother tincture is ∅. The abbreviation *MT* (*TM* in France) is also used to mean the same. Whilst some mother tinctures of low toxicity are used internally, these and others have external uses, when they may be applied directly, or in the form of creams, ointments, or lotions.

Bach flower remedies are similar to homoeopathic remedies, very safe, and are given in liquid dilution.

For administration by mouth, a *dose* is generally taken to mean: *one* pilule, one tablet, one coarse granule (globule), one small pinch of fine granules, one powder, or one drop of liquid potency, *irrespective of* the age or weight of the patient, and the designation of the remedy. *This notion of dosage will be taken as read throughout the text with regard to most remedies bearing a potency number*. It does *not* apply, however, to oral dosages of mother tinctures, herbal medicines, Bach flower remedies, minerals, and vitamins. For details on dosages of these preparations you are strongly advised to read Section 2 of this book.

The suggested quantities of remedy (one pilule, one tablet, etc.) are more than adequate to initiate or promote a *healing response* on the part of the body. Reinforcement of medicinal action is *not* achieved by giving larger amounts

4

than those stated. To do this would be wasteful, but not harmful.

An increase in medicinal effect must be produced by either dose repetition after a period of time, or by the use of higher potencies.

Let us consider the following prescription for *sun headache*, taken from the text:

Belladonna 30 2h

This states that, in an *average* case, one dose (i.e. one pilule, one tablet, etc.) of *Belladonna 30c* should be given initially every *two hours (2h)*. The strength of the treatment may be varied, however, according to the severity of the case. A mild case may require dosage repetition every *four hours (4h)*, and a severe case, every *hour (1h)*, or *half hour (½h)*. For the beginner, it is best to start with the directive of the text. Nevertheless, it should be noted that the frequency of repetition should be reduced as the patient improves, and in *most* instances the remedy should be *discontinued* once significant improvement has occurred.

Occasionally, after the administration of a remedy, the patient experiences what is termed *homoeopathic aggravation*. This is a transient worsening of the patient's symptoms, and may be caused by the use of too high a potency, or by too rapid dose repetition. In fact, it signifies *overstimulation* of the bodily healing response. Should this occur, the remedy should be *discontinued*, whereupon the phase of aggravation will be followed by one of remission, often proceeding to *cure*. However, it sometimes happens that this phase of remission is short-lived, and is followed by a resumption of the previous symptoms, although they are often less severe. In this case, the remedy should be reapplied, but less aggressively. Reduce the frequency of dosage, or select a lesser potency.

Throughout the text are indicated *average* potencies and repetition intervals. However, it is often the case that the traveller has the *right remedy*, but in the *wrong potency*. In this instance, the following **conversion guide** will be found helpful:

(1) The commonly prescribed potencies 6 and 30 are largely used throughout the text.

(2) A 6 should be given twice as often as a 30. Conversely, a 30 should be given half as often as a 6.

(3) A 30 should be given twice as often as a 200. Conversely, a 200 should be given half as often as a 30.

(4) Where the strength of the available remedy is other than 6, 30, or 200, take it to the nearest of these three elective potencies, e.g. a 9 should be treated as a 6. Should this elective potency be the same as that given in the text, the remedy should be applied in the same way. Should this elective potency be different from that stated in the text, then apply rules 2 and/or 3, given above.

Let us consider an example of these conversion rules in practice:

TEXT STATES: *Apis mellifica 6 2h*

AVAILABLE REMEDY: *Apis mellifica 100*

The nearest elective potency to the above is *30.*

A *30* should be given half as often as a *6.*

Therefore, the adjusted interval between doses is *four hours.*

The traveller's prescription will be:

Apis mellifica 100 4h

These conversion rules, whilst not strictly accurate, are a *practical approximation.* Whilst they may be freely applied to the *majority* of the prescriptions given in this book, there are certain *exceptions* where they are inappropriate, and these are stated in the text. Additionally, *it must not be assumed* that these rules apply to *all* homoeopathic prescribing. They most certainly would not be applicable to the treatment of common chronic diseases such as eczema, asthma, and arthritis, where the selection of potency is an *expert matter* to be reserved for the homoeopathic practitioner.

Under each section of the text, the traveller will observe that a number of *alternative* prescriptions is generally listed. Unless otherwise stated, it is important to choose but *one* prescription. Giving two or more prescriptions simultaneously, without expert knowledge, may result in *inimical or antidotal interactions* between the remedies concerned.

However, it may be assumed that *external and internal remedies may be combined usefully*.

The text *simplifies* the matter of remedy selection in four ways (or combinations of these):

(1) A single, most generally useful remedy is quoted.

(2) Several remedies are quoted, but their differential indications are given.

(3) Several remedies are quoted without differential indications, but they are listed in order of importance, the first quoted being that most frequently indicated.

(4) A *mixture* of known efficacy is quoted, or an acceptable *combination* of remedies is indicated.

Where a selection has been made, but the selected remedy is *unavailable*, choose the next alternative rather than do nothing.

Finally, some general advice on the *administration* of homoeopathic remedies:

(1) Pilules, tablets, and coarse granules (globules) should be sucked rather than swallowed (absorption is more reliable).

(2) Pilules, tablets, and coarse granules (globules) may be *inhaled by babies and unconscious people*. For such, remember to crush them to a fine powder before use. If you are using coarse granules, you will need several of them to generate a manageable quantity of powder for one dose. Alternatively, you may safely use fine granules or liquid potencies.

(3) All remedies should receive minimal direct handling. Do not put your fingers inside the vial.

(4) Ideally, the consumption of food and drink (and cleaning of teeth) should not occur 10 minutes before and after the oral administration of a remedy.

(5) Ideally, *no coffee*, decaffeinated or normal, should be taken during a course of homoeopathic treatment. Coffee tends to antidote the action of many remedies. However, tea, and alcohol in moderation are generally allowable.

(6) The homoeopathic prescriptions given in the text, where the remedy is followed by a potency number (e.g. *6*, *30*), are safe for patients on *orthodox drug therapies* from

their own physicians, with one exception. Alcohol is present in small quantities in homoeopathic preparations, but may produce adverse reactions in patients taking *Antabuse* therapy for alcoholism. Orthodox drug therapies should not be stopped without taking medical advice.

(7) Pilules, tablets, and granules are sugar-based. The amount of sugar ingested as a single dose is insufficient to adversely affect either diabetics or hypoglycaemics. However, patients who suffer from *disaccharide intolerance* should be restricted to the use of liquid potencies only.

(8) Whilst homoeopathic remedies are largely safe when given during *pregnancy and lactation*, certain rules should be observed. You are advised to consult *Section 8* of this book, entitled *For Women Travellers*.

(9) It is often necessary to interrupt the regularity of dosage of any medicine because of sleep. Recommence on waking.

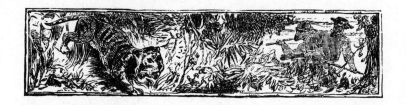

Section 2

PRESCRIBING TINCTURES, HERBS, AND SUNDRIES

In this section we consider the principles of prescribing for the remaining medicaments of the text.

External applications may contain homoeopathic mother tinctures, homoeopathic liquid potencies, herbal medicines, or vitamins. All those stated in the text are perfectly safe for use in pregnancy, lactation, and at all ages. Occasionally, however, allergic reactions do occur, with the production of a localised and itchy skin-rash. Should this occur, the application must be discontinued. Persons suffering from eczema are particularly prone to this type of reaction, and you are advised to test a small area of skin with the application before proceeding to more extensive use.

Bach flower remedies are given in great dilution, are non-toxic, and very safe at all ages, in pregnancy and lactation. Ask your homoeopathic pharmacist to prepare the appropriate dilution in alcohol, which will act as a preservative. The Bach remedies are not qualified by a potency number. The standard dose is *four drops*, given directly on to the tongue.

It is desirable not to eat, drink, or clean your teeth for ten minutes before or after administration. The dose is the same for all the Bach remedies, and at all ages. Undesirable side-effects are extremely rare, but patients taking *Antabuse* therapy for alcoholism should not take these remedies. Other orthodox drug therapies are compatible. Bach flower remedies are identified in the text by the use of the word *Bach* before the name of the remedy (e.g. *Bach Walnut*). They should be stored away from daylight and perfumed substances.

Homoeopathic *mother tinctures* are strong alcoholic extracts, usually of plant material, and some of low toxicity are recommended for internal use. The dose stated in the text (e.g. 5 drops) is the average *adult dose. This quantity should be reduced for children.* A good general rule is to give *one fifth of the stated adult dose for each 10kg (22lb) of weight.* For example, if the stated dose were *5 drops*, then the dose for a *30kg* child would be *3 drops*. It is generally advisable to take the prescribed dose in a little water to dilute the taste, which may be unpleasant. A few teaspoons of water will suffice. They may be taken on an empty stomach, or after food. Mother tinctures are not compatible with *Antabuse* therapy. Neither should they be used in pregnancy and lactation, nor along with orthodox drugs *without taking expert advice.* Side-effects are, however, relatively rare with regard to those tinctures mentioned in the text. Should they occur, they must be discontinued. Mother tinctures are identified in the text by the use of the symbol ø. They should be stored away from daylight. *It is important not to exceed the stated dose and dose frequency.*

The internal dosage of *minerals and vitamins* is quoted in milligrams (mg) or, in the case of vitamins, in international units (IU). Those stated represent average *adult* dosages, and should not be exceeded. For children, the dose should be *one fifth of the adult dose for each 10kg (22lb) of body weight.* Vitamins and minerals should only be taken in pregnancy on the advice of a physician. Those allergic to yeast should not take vitamins of the *B group.* Those with gall-bladder disease should not take oily supplements, such as *vitamin E capsules. Zinc* supplements may induce itching, or abdominal and muscular cramps. These side-effects are usually dose-related, and the prescribed dosage should be reduced to half.

We now come to the matter of *herbal (botanic) medicines*, concerning which a small number of useful prescriptions are given in the text. These should always be obtained from reliable sources, such as pharmacies and professional herbal establishments. To obtain the wrong herb or herbal preparation could have fatal consequences. The dose is expressed as a weight or a volume, and any special way of preparation (eg infusion) is described. The dose stated in the text is the average *adult dose*. For *children*, the dose must be reduced. Give *one fifth of the stated adult dose for every 10kg (22lb) of body weight*. It is important not to exceed the stated dosage, or calculated child's dosage, or prescribe more frequently than stated in the text. Whilst the herbal prescriptions that have been chosen may be regarded as reasonably safe in their appropriate dosage, they should not be taken in pregnancy and lactation, or in conjunction with orthodox drugs, without taking expert advice. Should any side-effects occur, they should be discontinued immediately. Herbalism, in terms of safety, must be considered to lie mid-way between homoeopathy and orthodox medicine.

All herbs and herbal preparations should be kept in well-sealed, dark or opaque containers. Ideally, they should be stored in a cool, dark, dry place. Dried herbs and herbal tablets are prone to go mouldy in hot and humid climates, but this may be prevented by placing *desiccant capsules* in their containers, which are readily obtained from any conventional pharmacy.

Remember that it is seldom necessary to wake a sleeping patient, except in the gravest cases, in order to preserve the regularity of administration of any medicine, be it homoeopathic, herbal, or otherwise. Recommencement of the dosage regime upon waking is generally acceptable, with little loss of efficacy.

G-6-PD deficiency

Persons with this inherited enzymatic deficiency should avoid all Bach or herbal preparations containing *vervain*, vitamin C supplements, and low potencies (less than *6c*, or *12x*) of the remedy *Caeruleum methylenum*, used in the prevention and treatment of bilharziasis. This matter will be of particular concern to black people, and those of Mediterranean origin. Please consult *Section 11* for further details, given under *Broad bean poisoning (Favism)*.

Keep all medicines out of the reach of children!

Table 2.1

Examples of common abbreviations used in homoeopathic pharmacy, and to be found in the text:

Abbreviation	Meaning
6	6th centesimal potency
6c	ditto
6 CH	ditto
6x	6th decimal potency
D6	ditto
6M	6000th centesimal potency (M = 1000c)
6h	to be given every 6 hours
6lb	6 pounds (avoirdupois)
6kg	6 kilograms (1kg = 2.2lb)
6g	6 grams (1000g = 1kg)
6mg	6 milligrams (1000mg = 1g)
6mcg (6μg)	6 micrograms (1000mcg = 1mg)
6ml	6 millilitres (1000ml = 1 litre)
	[1 level standard teaspoon = 5ml]
6IU (6iu)	6 international units
6gtt	6 drops
1gt	1 drop
ø	mother tincture
MT (TM)	ditto
aa (AA)	of each (in equal amounts)
qs	as much as suffices

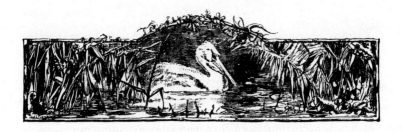

Section 3

IMMUNIZATION AND PREVENTION

The best form of infective disease prevention is *avoidance*!
Put simply:
   Avoid drinking contaminated water.
   Avoid cleaning your teeth in contaminated water.
   Avoid swimming in contaminated water.
   Avoid eating doubtful foods.
   Avoid being bitten.
   Avoid close physical contact with doubtful persons.
   Avoid walking bare-footed in some places.

Further details concerning these points will be given later.
For the moment, remember that *avoidance* is your *first*
friend, and immunization your second.

Ideally, the traveller should start thinking about immunization about six weeks prior to departure, in respect of which
there are two main categories of technique to be considered:
the *conventional*, and the *homoeopathic*.

The conventional technique usually involves the administration of inactivated, or attenuated live organisms, or
their products in order to induce the active production of
antibodies. It constitutes a crude form of homoeopathy.

Administration is generally by injection, but may be via the oral route (see: polio). Alternatively, *passive immunity* may be conferred by the injection of human antibody material (see: hepatitis A). The level of immunity conferred, the side-effects, and medical contraindications are well-documented with regard to the conventional method. Some vaccines produce poor immunity (eg cholera vaccine). Some may involve a slight risk to the foetus when given during pregnancy. Each vaccine must be assessed individually with respect to its benefits and problems.

The homoeopathic technique usually consists of the *oral* administration of a remedy prepared in *great dilution* from the offending bacterium or virus. Such a remedy prepared from a microorganism is termed a *nosode*. Those nosodes utilized for immunization, correctly given, are immensely safe, virtually free from side-effects, and may be given in pregnancy and lactation. Alternatively, a remedy other than a nosode may be given preventatively which would be used to treat the disease in question (eg malaria). Such remedies are also generally very safe. Safety and lack of side-effects thus characterise the homoeopathic method. Homoeopathic remedies would seem to work by actively stimulating the immune system of the body in some way. The manner in which this occurs, however, has not been totally elucidated.

Whilst the value of homoeopathic remedies in the *treatment* of disease has been well-established, their use in the field of immunization has been, as yet, incompletely documented. There is, however, considerable evidence of their action in the control of the spread of epidemics, but this in itself, for the present, cannot justify a total elimination of the conventional approach.

Bearing these facts in mind, the homoeopathic technique of immunization is strongly recommended in the following situations:

(1) Where the conventional technique is of poor statistical efficacy (see: cholera). Homoeopathic remedies may be given in substitution, or, alternatively, may be used to complement the orthodox method.

(2) Where a conventional immunization course has not been completed. This situation generally arises when a last-minute decision has been made to journey abroad. Homoeopathic remedies may be used to complement the orthodox approach.

(3) Where there is no satisfactory conventional technique (see: bacillary dysentery), or where there is lack of availability of conventional technique (as in remote places).

(4) Where there are strong medical contraindications to orthodox immunization.

(5) Where the traveller, whether from a dislike of injections or lack of trust in orthodoxy, refuses the conventional approach.

Should the homoeopathic method be selected, it is important to realise that the immunity conferred by a single dose of remedy is *short-lived*. Doses must be repeated at regular intervals (often once weekly) in order to produce the required effect, and this regular repetition, which should ideally commence about two weeks prior to departure, should be continued for the duration of the period of infective risk. It is totally inadequate to rely on a short course of three doses, which would be but a vain attempt to emulate conventional immunization. A reduction in the frequency of dose repetition is only justified if side-effects occur regularly after each dose. These rarities, in any event, are of a minor nature (e.g. mild diarrhoea), but suggest that the interval between doses should be initially doubled. Alternatively, a lesser potency might be selected (but never less than *6c* or *12x*). It is to be emphasised, however, that such modifications to dosage are rarely required.

Apart from their direct use in immunization, homoeopathic remedies are of value in reducing the ill-effects of the conventional technique. Injections are painful, and many, especially children, find them singularly upsetting. There may also be severe local or general reactions (inflammation, swelling, fever, etc.). Although a relatively rare phenomenon, the onset of chronic disease in some individuals is attributable to a previous immunization injection (this is termed *miasmic disease*).

15

To reduce the severity of injection pain, and calm the sensitive, give the following 30 minutes before, and immediately after the procedure:

Chamomilla 30

To reduce the local reaction, the general reaction, and the likelihood of miasmic disease, give the following remedy, commencing on the morning of the injection:

Thuja 30 12h for 3 days (6 doses)

Chamomilla and *Thuja* are compatible with each other. *Thuja* does not interfere with the generation of active immunity.

Let us now consider the available conventional and homoeopathic immunization techniques in greater detail (further documentation of the relevant diseases will be given later in the text):

Typhoid   Section 23

The basic conventional programme of immunization consists of two injections separated by an interval of 4 to 6 weeks, with the generation of reasonable immunity for a period of 3 years. The efficacy of the technique is, however, not 100%, and is diminished by subsequent exposure to a large dose of typhoid bacteria. A single injection, moreover, only confers 70–80% immunity for a period of 1 year. The method is not recommended for infants under one year of age, or those suffering from an acute fever (eg influenza), and should only be considered cautiously in pregnancy. Persons who have been repeatedly immunized in this way, especially if they are above 35 years of age, are particularly prone to severe reactions to this technique. The use of *Thuja*, as documented above, is strongly indicated in such circumstances. Two new vaccines are now available. Typhim V is given as a single injection, but should not be used in those under 18 months of age, and in pregnancy. Vivotif is a course of three capsules of live attenuated virus, which should not be given in pregnancy, to children less than 6 years of age, to those with gastrointestinal upset, and those with a suppressed immune system.

Homoeopathically, take *Salmonella typhi nosode 30 once weekly*.

Paratyphoid   *Section 23*
No conventional method of immunization is now available. An alternative approach is to take *Salmonella paratyphi AB nosode 30 once weekly*.

Cholera   *Section 10*
The conventional method of immunization consists of two injections separated by an interval of 7 to 28 days, with booster injections being given every 6 months. The technique, however, is surprisingly ineffective, and has a 50% failure rate. Indeed, the World Health Organisation (WHO) no longer recommends its routine use for travellers to or from cholera-infected areas. Nevertheless, certain countries still require written proof of orthodox cholera immunization before entry is permitted. Conventional immunization should not be given to those who have experienced a previous severe reaction to the vaccine, or those suffering from an acute fever (eg influenza). It should be prescribed cautiously in pregnancy. Repeated use of the vaccine may result in the production of a severe generalised reaction.

Homoeopathically, take *Vibrio cholerae nosode 30 once weekly* (for another method, see *Section 10*). Remember, however, that cholera is a classic example of a disease where *avoidance* is more important than immunization; that is to say, the avoidance of *contaminated food and drink*. The same might be said of typhoid, paratyphoid, hepatitis A, and dysentery.

Hepatitis A   *Section 24*
Passive immunization is available in the form of an injection of human normal immunoglobulin (immune protein). This should be applied with caution in pregnancy. Effective immunity lasts approximately 4 months. An injectable vaccine, producing long-lasting active immunity, is now available for those over 16 years of age.

Homoeopathically, consider *Hepatitis A nosode 30 once weekly*.

Hepatitis B   Section 24
This is not a disease that should concern the average travel-ler. Unlike hepatitis A, which is largely communicated via poor food hygiene, hepatitis B is contracted via sexual con-tact, poor surgical technique, unsterile injection methods, unsterile acupuncture, and tattooing. Additionally, there is a possibility, though unproven, that this disease may be acquired from biting insects, such as bed-bugs. Orthodox immunization techniques by injection, producing either active or passive immunity, are available for high-risk groups.

Homoeopathically, *Hepatitis B nosode 30 once weekly* might be considered.

Yellow fever   Section 24
Conventional immunization, which is *almost* 100% effective, is given as a single injection, and confers immunity for a period of at least 10 years. The vaccine should not be given to those with an acute fever (eg influenza), those with certain types of cancer, people taking high doses of steroids, people on immune suppressive therapy, those who are receiving radiotherapy, those who are allergic to eggs or certain anti-biotics (neomycin or polymyxin), and AIDS positive indi-viduals. It should be considered with caution in pregnancy, and in children under 9 months of age. An international certificate of vaccination is required by some countries.

Homoeopathically, take *Yellow fever nosode 30 once weekly*. Whatever you do, take measures to *avoid* being bitten by the mosquitoes which transmit this serious disease.

Malaria   Section 20
No true immunization technique is available, but orally administered orthodox drugs can be taken to reduce the chances of contracting the disease. These must be continued for 4–8 weeks *after* return from a malaria zone. Even so, they are no better than 85% effective in the prevention of malaria, and some of these drugs should not be given in

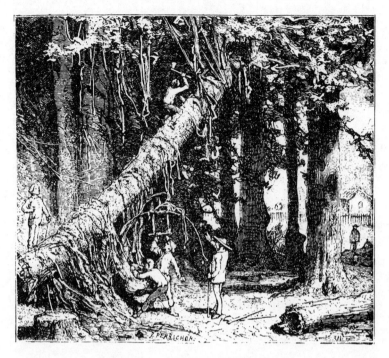

Gathering Peruvian bark for quinine

pregnancy. Indeed, the situation with regard to the development of resistance by malarial parasites to orthodox preventative medicines is now of some gravity. Responsibility for this accelerating disaster must largely be taken by the medical profession itself, the origin of which is comparable to the generation of bacterial resistance from the misuse and over-prescription of antibiotics. The giving of valuable preventative drugs to a multitude of individuals, without any advice on the prevention of mosquito bites, has allowed the malarial parasites more than adequate opportunity to produce resistant mutations; more importantly so, that species which causes the potentially fatal 'malignant' variety of the disease. In this respect, particularly dangerous areas are Thailand and neighbouring countries, Central and South America, Kenya, and sub-Saharan Africa. Recent research into the use of the Chinese herb *Artemisia apiacea*, a type

19

of wormwood, appears promising, but, if abused, will no doubt suffer the same fate as the current orthodox drugs. Interestingly enough, another variety of wormwood, *Artemisia absinthium*, has properties suggesting its possible homoeopathic use in the prevention and treatment of cerebral malaria.

Avoidance of mosquito bites is obviously of the greatest importance in the prevention of this disease, despite the availability of antimalarial drugs (see Section 14).

Even if you are taking orthodox preventative medication, you should seriously consider taking the appropriate homoeopathic remedies as well. The following combined regime should be taken, preferably from 2 weeks before travelling, until 6 weeks after return from endemic malarial areas:

(1) *Malaria officinalis 30, one dose morning and evening on a single named day each week (eg Saturday)*

(2) On the remaining 6 days of each week, take:
   Cinchona officinalis 8x 12h
   [where this potency is unavailable, use *6–30 12h*]

Polio (Poliomyelitis) Section 24

Both conventional oral and injection techniques are available for the prevention of this disease, with the production of highly effective active immunity. There is, however, a small but definite risk of contracting the disease itself as a result of taking oral polio vaccine (approximately 1 in 2 million in the United Kingdom). Poliomyelitis is a serious hazard for travellers to developing countries, good hygiene alone not guaranteeing protection.

Homoeopathically, the traveller might consider *Poliomyelitis nosode 30 once weekly*.

Tetanus Section 15

The risk of contracting this disease, which occurs as the result of wound contamination, is increased in the case of certain activities. These include: trekking, exploring, and mountaineering. Correct wound cleansing diminishes the risk. Highly effective orthodox immunization techniques are available.

Homoeopathically, consider either *Clostridium tetani nosode 30 once weekly*, or *Ledum 30 12h*.

Bacillary dysentery (Shigellosis)   *Section 10*
No orthodox immunization technique is available. Scrupulous food and drink hygiene is of the utmost importance in its prevention. The administration of *Shigella co. nosode 30 once weekly* may be helpful. As with *travellers' diarrhoea* in general, the use of the remedy *Crataegus* may also contribute some protection (see *Section 10*).

Diphtheria   *Section 22*
The acquisition of this disease may be considered a serious risk to travellers in *developing* countries. Many adults are, however, immune to this. The traveller's immune status with respect to diphtheria is established by the Schick skin test. Orthodox immunization by injection is available, but should be avoided during acute fevers (eg influenza), and should only be used with caution during pregnancy. Diphtheria of the skin can be largely avoided by thorough skin hygiene.

Homoeopathically, consider *Diphtherinum 30 once weekly*.

Meningococcal meningitis   *Section 23*
The prevention of this serious disease is largely of concern to those who travel to the so-called *meningitis belt* of Africa, Nepal, New Delhi, and Mecca. Since spread is via exhaled droplets, avoidance in these areas may be impossible. Orthodox immunization technique by injection is available, but should be avoided during acute fevers (eg influenza), and considered cautiously in pregnancy.

Homoeopathically, consider *Neisseria meningitidis co. nosode 30 once weekly*.

Rabies   *Section 15*
This disease is usually contracted as the result of an animal bite. Correct cleansing of the wound is of the utmost impor-

21

tance in its prevention. Orthodox pre-exposure immunization by injection is available for high-risk travellers, such as zoologists, hunters, explorers, and botanists. It should not, however, be used for low-risk travellers, since rare but serious side-effects have been reported. Conventional post-exposure immunization techniques by injection are also available for those who have been bitten, and must be considered as highly important in disease prevention.

Where conventional pre-exposure immunization is unavailable, *Hydrophobinum 30 once weekly* may be considered. Where conventional post-exposure immunization is unavailable, consider *Hydrophobinum 30 once daily for at least 4 months*.

Japanese B encephalitis   Section 24
This disease is transmitted to man by the bite of a calicine mosquito found in the rice fields of South East Asia and the Far East. It mainly occurs during the monsoon season. Avoidance of areas where rice cultivation and pig farming co-exist largely removes the risk of contracting this disease. An orthodox immunization technique to prevent this disease is available, but is unnecessary for short-stay travellers who avoid high-risk areas.

Homoeopathically, consider *Japanese B encephalitis nosode 30 once weekly*.

European tick-borne encephalitis   Section 24
This disease is transmitted to man by the bite of an infected tick found in warm forested parts of Central Europe and Scandinavia, especially in areas of heavy undergrowth. Those mainly at risk are, therefore, hikers, campers, hunters, biologists, geologists, and foresters. Careful avoidance of tick bites is the best means of prevention. An orthodox preventative immunization technique is also available.

Homoeopathically, consider *European tick-borne encephalitis nosode 30 once weekly*.

Plague   Section 23
This disease is transmitted to humans via the bites of fleas carried by various rodents. *The best defence is avoidance.*

Avoid rodents found in plague areas, such as rats, rabbits, chipmunks, and squirrels. Avoid contact with animal carcasses found on expeditions in plague areas. Use insect repellents, particularly on the legs and clothing. Use insecticides, and rodenticides at resting places. Regularly apply anti-flea preparations to domestic pets in risk areas.

Orthodox immunization techniques, by injection, are available for those at special risk, but are not necessary for the average traveller. Their efficacy, however, is less than 100%, and they should be avoided in pregnancy.

Homoeopathically, consider *Yersinia pestis nosode 30 once weekly.*

Typhus *Section 25*
See *Section 25* for a description of the various types of this disease, and their corresponding modes of transmission. Vaccines have been produced for the prevention of various types of typhus in high risk personnel. These may be difficult to obtain, and some have become unavailable. No effective vaccine has been produced for scrub typhus, where the orthodox method involves the use of prophylactic antibiotics.

Homoeopathically, the use of specific nosodes may be considered, such as *Scrub typhus nosode 30 once weekly.*

Bilharziasis
See Section 21

Lyme disease
See Section 14

Dengue *Section 24*
An effective vaccine against this mosquito-borne disease has been developed, but is not commercially available.

Homoeopathically, consider *Dengue nosode 30 once weekly.*

When it has been determined that several homoeopathic preventative remedies should be taken on a weekly basis, where possible it is advantageous to take them as a single dose each week, in the form of a mixture especially prepared by your homoeopathic pharmacist. Try to take your preventative remedies on a specified day of the week, at a particular time (eg 10 minutes before breakfast). If you forget, take them later rather than not. Even if other homoeopathic or conventional treatments are required for the treatment of illness, the preventative regime should be continued. Remember, however, that poor general health, hygiene or nutrition will weaken the preventative aspects of the remedies. Similarly, it would appear that the use of conventional antibiotics is often antidotal to the action of homoeopathic remedies in general.

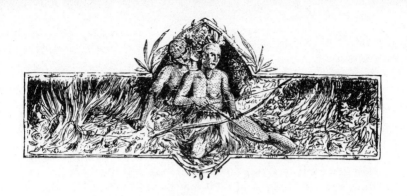

Section 4

TRAVELLERS' NERVES

Many trips are spoilt by nervous disorders associated with travelling, such as anxiety, fear, and insomnia. Even before the journey has begun, such psychological problems may become manifest. Those who are absent from home for a prolonged period may suffer from what I have termed *immigrant syndrome* (see below). Homoeopathic remedies can do much to alleviate these disorders of the mind, without the drugging effect associated with orthodox tranquillisers and antidepressants.

Anticipatory nerves: apprehension
Anxiety concerning journey or destination may be either rational or irrational. A satisfactory prescription may be based upon the way in which the nervous state manifests itself:

(1) Overtalkative, cannot rest, busy with many tasks (a picture of *overactivity*):

Argentum nitricum 30 4h

(2) Lethargic, motionless, *silent* (a picture of *under-activity*):

> *Gelsemium 30 4h*

Whichever remedy is selected as more appropriate, persons of a generally nervous disposition may find the 30th potency too strong for them, in that it may produce a transient aggravation of their symptoms. Such persons should consider commencing treatment with a lower potency (eg 6). Conversely, generally non-anxious individuals, who suffer extreme apprehension of travel, may require higher potencies (eg 200), in order to allay their anxieties. In either case, the initial dosage interval is as stated above (4h).

Anticipatory nerves: fear
The above remedies will be ineffective where the dominant mental state is one of *fear*. Great fear, dread, fears death may be at hand, terror, *panic*:

(1) *Aconite 30 2h*
(2) *Bach Rescue Remedy 1h*

Anticipatory nerves: overexcitement
Some people become so overexcited about a trip that they cannot rest. They present a picture which resembles that given above for *Argentum nitricum* (see *apprehension*). They are, however, not dreading the trip, but are, indeed, *looking forward* to it. In this situation a different remedy is indicated:

> *Coffea cruda 30 12h*

Homesickness

(1) *Capsicum 30 12h*
(2) *Bach Honeysuckle 6h*

Inadaptability
General inadaptability to change:

> *Bach Walnut 6h*

Immigrant syndrome

A combination of homesickness, inadaptability, and a sense of isolation, arising from emigration or prolonged absence from home. Consider the following two remedies given in combination:

> *Bach Walnut* +
> *Bach Honeysuckle 6h*

Sensitivity to noise & smells

Especially in irritable and precise people:

> *Nux vomica 30 6h*

Sensitivity to noise

(1) Intolerance of the *slightest* noise:

> *Theridion 30 6h*

(2) Intolerance of *loud* noise:

> *Borax 30 6h*

Sensitivity to tobacco smoke

Especially useful in bars and cafés:

> *Ignatia 30 2h*

Aversion to crowded places

Also known as *agoraphobia*. Consider:

> *Argentum nitricum 30 6h*

Persons of a generally nervous disposition may find that potencies lower than 30 may suit them better (eg 6), in that a transient aggravation of symptoms may occur with higher potencies.

Impatience

Excessive impatience and anger when being kept waiting, or when subjected to the shortcomings of others:

(1) *Bach Impatiens 6h*
(2) *Nux vomica 30 6h*

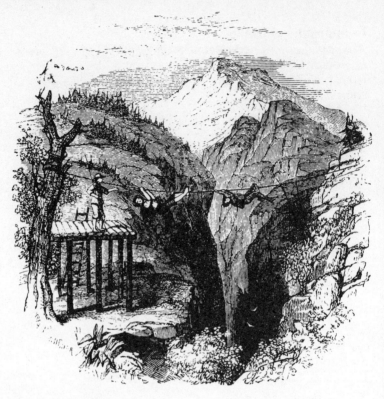

Nervous exhaustion

From generally overdoing things, or too many late nights:

(1) *Kali phosphoricum 6 6h*
(2) *Panax ginseng 6 12h*

Fractious children

Many small children, much to the distress of their parents, become extremely difficult as the result of travelling. Usually this results from disturbance of their usual routine. Consider:

(1) Restless, spiteful, cross, irritable, whining, unco-operative, but with a *desire to be carried or petted, which improves the mood*:

Chamomilla 30 2h

(2) Similar to the former, but *does not wish to be touched, carried, or even looked at:*

> *Cina 30 2h*

Psychological problems of flight

See Section 5

Travellers' Insomnia

I have left the consideration of sleeplessness to the last, since its homoeopathic treatment will depend upon the cause, and the main causes have been discussed above. Insomnia from overexcitement will thus be treated differently from that due to noise sensitivity. The treatment cited for the cause will treat the associated sleep problem. Additionally, however, you might like to consider the following:

(1) Sleeplessness due to mind being full of thoughts (especially pleasant ones):

> *Coffea cruda 200, a single dose at bed-time*

(2) Early waking due to alcoholic or gastronomic over-indulgence:

> *Nux vomica 200, a single dose at bed-time*

(3) Mild sleep-inducing herbal tablets are available commercially (from pharmacies and health-food stores), which may be taken irrespective of cause. By way of example, the contents of a typical proprietary tablet are as follows:

Valeriana (Valerian) dried extract 160mg
Humulus lupulus (Hops) dried extract 200mg
Passiflora incarnata (Passion flower) dried extract 130mg
The adult dose is stated as *2 tablets swallowed at bed-time.*
They are best avoided in pregnancy or lactation.

(4) Some sleep better upon a pillow filled with dried hops (*Humulus lupulus*). The aroma of the hops induces sleep in mild cases of insomnia.

(5) See also *Jet-lag (Section 5)*.

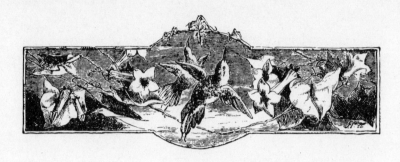

Section 5

PROBLEMS OF FLIGHT

The increasing use of the aeroplane as a means of transportation gives rise to many problems for the traveller, against which homoeopathic remedies may be taken with good effect. These problems may be either psychological or physical.

Anticipatory nerves
Apprehension, fear, or overexcitement:

See Section 4

Fear of heights
More commonly experienced in small aircraft. Consider:

Argentum nitricum 30 4h

Fear of descent
Dread of the descent for landing, or the sudden descent associated with *air pockets*:

Borax 30 4h

Claustrophobia

Fear of restriction to a confined space. The same is occasionally experienced by railway travellers, and pot-holers. Consider:

Argentum nitricum 30 4h

Jet-lag

The speedy transportation of the modern traveller by jet across the time-zones of the World generates this phenomenon. The biological clock mechanism is unable to adapt with sufficient rapidity to the new time of the destination. This results in disturbance of sleep pattern, excessive fatigue, difficulty in concentration, and disturbance of appetite and bowel movement patterns. Left untreated, it takes approximately one day for each time zone traversed for recovery to occur, although it is true to say that westward travel is often better tolerated than eastward. Fortunately, however, adaptation of the biological clock can be accelerated by the homoeopathic method. The following remedy should be taken regularly for a period *from two days before to three days after the flight*:

Cocculus indicus 30 12h

The same prescription will be found of use for *any prolonged journey, with disturbance of normal sleeping pattern*. If, however, the administration of the above remedy is delayed until *after* the flight or journey, it may induce some degree of oversleeping.

Swollen feet (Postural oedema/edema)

This is promoted by immobility, and is more common in women, especially the elderly. It may be reduced by frequent walks along the gangway of the plane, but this is not always an easy matter, especially in smaller aircraft. The same problem may be associated with coach and railway journeys. Even if the occasional walk does little to alleviate swelling of the feet, it does much to prevent the development of serious clots in the deep veins of the legs (deep vein thrombosis), which could have a fatal outcome. A useful

31

homoeopathic prescription to prevent foot swelling, which should be commenced 24 hours before travelling, is as follows:

> Urtica urens ø 5 drops 6h

Earache and sinus pain (Barotrauma)

Earache upon *descent*, known as *otic barotrauma or aero-otitis*, is an extremely common phenomenon. As a plane descends, the pressure within increases, leading to contraction of the air contained in the middle ear. Should the eustachian tube, which connects the middle ear chamber to the throat, be blocked, the eardrum will become indrawn, and severe pain will be experienced. Such obstruction is common in catarrhal patients, whether the catarrh be a long-term problem or in the form of an acute catarrh, such as the common cold. A similar phenomenon, termed *sinus barotrauma*, may occur with blocked sinuses, leading to intense pain in the cheeks, or above the eyes. The sinus variety is, however, less common than the otic. A useful physical treatment for both types is the so-called *Valsalva manoeuvre*, the objective of which is to force air into the middle ear cavities or sinuses:

> *Pinch your nostrils tightly shut with finger & thumb.*
> *Take a deep breath & hold it.*
> *Seal your lips tightly together.*
> *Forcefully breath out, so as to blow out your cheeks.*
> *Repeat several times.*
> *Popping sounds signify success.*

Other physical methods recommended for inflating the eustachian tubes (but not the sinuses) include:

> *Wiggling the jaw from side to side.*
> *Opening the jaw wide.*
> *Swallowing, assisted by sucking a boiled sweet.*
> *Swallowing whilst pinching the nostrils tightly.*

Obviously, any treatment instituted to improve the catarrhal state before departure will reduce the likelihood of barotrauma, and for this matter you should enlist the services of an homoeopathic practitioner or acupuncturist. However, this point aside, the homoeopathic method now given may be regarded as useful in a large number of cases as a short-term preventative against barotrauma in those predisposed to it:

> *On the day before departure, in the morning, take a single dose of Medorrhinum 200 (or 30).*
> *12 hours later take one more dose of Medorrhinum 200 (or 30).*
> *From the morning of the day of departure take Borax 30 6h, until landing.*

The remedy *Medorrhinum* should not be given in pregnancy and lactation, without taking proper advice. In such circumstances, or where the remedy has not been obtained, commence *Borax 30 6h from the morning of the day before departure.*

If your trip is less than 14 days, do not repeat the *Medorrhinum* before the return flight. Merely take the *Borax* as described in the previous paragraph.

Toothache (Aero-odontalgia)

Pain in a tooth on *ascent* is a rare occurrence, but may signify that the pulp (nerve) of the tooth is heavily infected. It is due to the expansion of gas within the pulp chamber. The pain improves upon descent. Remember to seek urgent dental attention on arrival at your destination, but, as emergency treatment during flight, consider:

(1) *Apis mellifica 30 1h*
(2) *Coffea cruda 30 1h*

Additionally, holding *cold or iced* water in the mouth may help, by inducing contraction of the pulpal gas.

Flatulence (Wind)

As a modern pressurised aircraft ascends, so the pressure within it drops from approximately 760mmHg to 600mmHg. This reduction of pressure causes gases within the gut of the passenger to expand, which may lead to a feeling of abdominal distention and discomfort. Such a sensation will be exacerbated by tight clothing and belts, the consumption of fermentable foods, such as greens and beans, and the consumption of alcohol and carbonated drinks. In order to feel comfortable, it is, therefore, important to dress, eat, and drink appropriately. Additionally, homoeopathic remedies may be taken to improve the state of comfort:

(1) For upper abdominal distention:

Carbo vegetabilis 30 2h

(2) For lower abdominal distention:

Lycopodium 6 2h

(3) For generalised abdominal distention:

Cinchona officinalis 30 2h

Further hazards of reduced cabin pressure
There are certain surgical conditions which may be adversely affected by the reduced cabin pressure discussed above. These include: recent abdominal, chest, cranial or ear operations; recent bleeding from the gut, collapsed lung, skull fractures, and plaster casts. Any traveller for whom these matters are relevant should consult his doctor before flying. The plaster cast, for example, which is not an uncommon sight on return flights from skiing resorts, contains trapped air. Upon exposure to the lower pressure of ascent, this will expand, and may cause compression of the limb and restriction of blood flow. For long flights, it may be considered necessary to split the cast. Passengers with hernias should be issued with a truss, especially if flying in unpressurised aircraft.

Hypoxia (Lack of oxygen)
Associated with the reduced pressure on ascent, even in modern pressurised aircraft, is reduction in oxygen pressure. This leads to a small reduction of oxygen in the blood. For most travellers, this effect goes unnoticed. However, symptoms of *hypoxia* may develop in heavy smokers, those who have overindulged in alcohol, fatigued passengers, and those with heavy colds. These symptons, which are subtle in onset, resemble alcoholic intoxication, with the development of

confusion, disorientation, unsteadiness, and personality change, and are accompanied by a blueness of lips, nail beds, and ear lobes. Oxygen should be administered in such circumstances. Passengers particularly at risk are those suffering from certain major medical problems. These include: respiratory disease (such as chronic bronchitis and emphysema), heart disease (such as angina), anaemia (haemoglobin less than 9g/dl), and impairment of blood supply to the brain (as in stroke patients). Such passengers may not only develop the symptoms of hypoxia described above, but may also experience a worsening of their pre-existing condition. The chronic bronchitic may become more breathless, and the angina sufferer may experience chest pain. Oxygen, therefore, which is readily available on board, may well be required. Moreover, epileptic travellers may require additional medication for flying, in order to avoid seizures brought on by hypoxia. All these risk groups should avoid flying in *unpressurised* aircraft above 2000 metres, and, in any event, should always consult their physicians *before any flight*.

Dehydration

The air within the modern aircraft is extremely dry. As has been stated above, the worst thing is to fill yourself with alcoholic and carbonated drinks. Stick to fruit juices, uncarbonated spring water, and tea. If you wear contact lenses, beware! Contact lenses dry out whilst flying with great rapidity. An additional hazard is the insecticide aerosol. Shut your eyes whilst the cabin staff are spraying, to avoid the deposition of aerosol droplets on your contact lenses, with consequent eye irritation.

Airsickness

Since the modern aircraft usually flies above the worst turbulence, the matter of travel-sickness is irrelevant to most passengers. However, those who are particularly prone to this disorder should consult *Section 6*.

Pregnancy and flight

See Section 8

Pacemakers

Travellers fitted with cardiac pacemakers should be wary with regard to electromagnetic security screening systems in non-western countries. The matter should be explained to the local security officials, who will then carry out a personal body check as an alternative.

Air passengers' back

Prolonged immobility whilst flying may lead to the development or worsening of lumbago or sciatica:

See Section 7

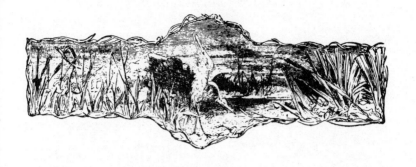

Section 6

TRAVEL-SICKNESS

Also known as *motion sickness*, this is an acute disorder associated with travelling, and is characterised by pallor, dizziness, sweating, abdominal discomfort, salivation, nausea, and finally vomiting. It is extremely common in children, who fortunately usually grow out of it. Cars and boats constitute the worst offenders in this respect. Modern passenger aircraft are seldom a problem (see *Airsickness, Section 5*). Bicycles are the safest.

Apart from motion, there are various visual and psychological causative factors. Certainly, heavy or greasy meals should be avoided before or during the journey. Discomfort and inconvenience aside, there are seldom any serious effects from this disorder. However, for diabetics on insulin it may be a major problem, and cause the blood sugar level to drop (*hypoglycaemia*). Neither does persistent vomiting do any good to the foetus in early pregnancy in women prone to miscarriage. Gastric ulcer patients may bleed from the lining of the stomach. Persistent vomiting in any patient will eventually produce dehydration, and attempts to rehydrate orally will usually fail until all vomiting has ceased. Conventional antihistamines may be administered to prevent or treat this disorder, but many have

37

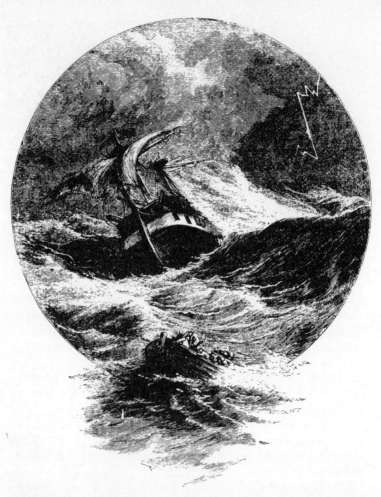

side-effects, including drowsiness and dry mouth, whilst drugs in pregnancy are, in any event, a bad idea. Additionally, in established travel-sickness, antihistamines are likely to be vomited up, rather than being retained and absorbed.

Fortunately, however, homoeopathic remedies come to the rescue of many people afflicted with travel-sickness, or a predisposition to it, without causing the drowsiness and dryness of the mouth associated with orthodox drugs:

(1) The following prescription is best used preventatively, although it may also be used for treatment of established travel-sickness. For maximum efficacy, in the case of a prolonged trip, treatment should begin *two days before travelling*. In the case of a short journey, such as a day's outing, the first dose should be given *not less than 1 hour prior to departure*. This prescription is a mixture of three homoeopathic remedies:

> *Cocculus indicus 30 +*
> *Petroleum 6 +*
> *Tabacum 6 6h*

If the remedy is supplied, as it usually is, in the form of tablets, pilules or coarse granules, and is being used to treat established travel-sickness, then it is best for the sufferer to crunch the remedy between his teeth in order to promote rapid oral absorption. Alternatively, crush the remedy to a fine powder before administration.

(2) Where the above mixture is unavailable, this single remedy will be of use in many cases, and should be administered similarly:

> *Cocculus indicus 30 6h*

(3) As an alternative, the following remedy may be used for both prevention and treatment. It is very safe, highly effective, and remarkably rapid in action. Whatever the length or nature of the proposed journey, a dose given even minutes before departure can be highly effective in the prevention of travel-sickness. The disadvantages are its unpleasant taste (to some), it feels hot as it is swallowed, and it requires the availability of clean water to dilute it. It is still to be highly recommended:

> *Zingiber ø 5–10 drops 2h*

For maximum effect, it is important not to over-dilute the drops. About 1 teaspoonful (5ml) of water will suffice for this dose. Remember to reduce the number of drops given to small children (see *Section 2*), and to reduce the quantity of water used proportionately.

Having satisfactorily controlled a bout of travel-sickness, the sufferer must be rehydrated slowly. Sips of water only – not large glassfuls!

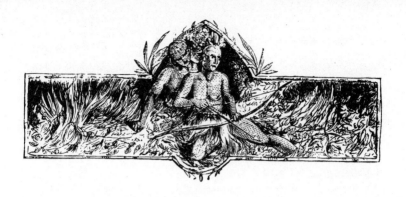

Section 7

TRAVELLERS' SPINE

Spinal problems associated with travelling, holidays, and working abroad are not at all uncommon. Often they are no more than an aggravation of an existing spinal disorder. The back, after all, is one of the more neglected parts of the human body. The teeth, eyes, and blood pressure are often checked with great regularity, the car does not escape its appropriate service, and yet the back receives little attention until it *breaks down*. On holiday, the breakdown of a spine may well be more catastrophic than the breakdown of your vehicle. It follows, therefore, that those who have any history of back or neck problems should consult a practitioner of osteopathy or chiropractic *before they travel*. When such disorders do arise on a trip, *homoeopathic remedies* will be found helpful to reduce pain, muscle spasm, inflammation, and stiffness. It must be emphasised, however, that they may not be totally curative in their own right, and that the services of an *osteopath* or *chiropractor* should be sought, to whose treatment the remedies are complementary. *Acupuncture* also may be highly effective in treating such cases, especially if combined with manipulation, but you should be certain that the practitioner, especially in developing countries, uses only properly sterilized needles. If this matter cannot be confirmed, it is better to suffer than to risk contracting either *Hepatitis B* or *AIDS*. Once some improvement has been obtained by the use of homoeopathic remedies, or the other methods described, remember that *gentle movement* is generally better than complete rest.

Lumbago

This term simply means backache of muscular or spinal origin. There may be spasm of the back muscles, with or without bruising, a sprain (tearing of fibres) of muscles or ligaments, minor but painful dislocations of vertebral joints, pressure on spinal nerves, or reactive inflammation. In the disorder known as *slipped disk*, the cushioning disk between two vertebrae is disrupted, and the disk material presses on spinal nerves, causing great pain. Great pain, however, is not diagnostic of this condition, and most cases of lumbago have a less serious origin. The homoeopathic treatment will be determined in part by the circumstances under which the condition arose, but mainly by the particular symptoms experienced.

The stiff back

Immobility whilst travelling is a frequent cause of lumbago. Air travel, long car journeys, and coach trips are common offenders. The smoothness of modern transportation is, in a sense, disadvantageous. The spine of the immobile passenger receives very little transmitted energy from the movement of the vehicle, a certain amount of passive movement of the spinal joints being valuable in the prevention of discomfort. Incorrect seating, with lack of an appropriate support for the sacral area at the bottom of the spine, or restriction of leg room, is also contributory. Obviously, regular trips along the gangway of the plane or coach, or frequent stops along the road would do much to prevent problems, but such active exercise is not always feasible.

Lacking both active and passive exercise, the passenger's back may become progressively more stiff and painful. Where the back feels *stiff*, is worse on initial movement and *better for continued movement*, which is generally the case with lumbago from immobility, consider taking the remedy that follows. Indeed, this remedy is useful in many cases of lumbago, irrespective of causation, where the patient loosens up with continued exercise:

(1) *Rhus toxicodendron 30 6h*

[here, the 30th potency is often vastly more effective than the 6th taken more frequently]

Whilst generally highly effective, the above remedy may fail in those travellers with a history of back weakness or recurrent lumbago. In such circumstances, and again *where the back is worse on initial movement and better for continued motion*, the following remedy should be considered:

(2) *Calcarea fluorica 6 6h*

[sometimes, potencies higher than 6 will cause temporary aggravation]

The bruised back
Let us now consider another situation with regard to travelling. The passenger is confined to his seat, but the journey is *rough or bumpy*. Cross-country trips, unmade roads, stiff car suspension, hard seats, or rough seas may be causative. Whilst, as I have stated, a certain amount of passive movement of the spine is desirable, excessive transmitted forces are deleterious. Here the back will often feel *bruised* rather than stiff, because of the spinal trauma. Yet, getting out of the seat and exercising will improve matters. Where the back feels *bruised*, but *improves with continued motion*, which is often the case in lumbago from rough journeys, the following remedy is well indicated. Indeed, it may be used in the case of lumbago from any cause, provided that these characteristic symptoms are present. It may, for example, be found useful for *campers' backache*, from sleeping on hard ground, which frequently has similar features:

Bellis perennis 30 6h

The strained back
Lifting and carrying heavy suitcases, haversacks or shopping bags, and indulging in more exercise than usual, such as

tennis, golf and gardening, are common causes of this problem. Where the lumbago is of *mild to moderate* severity, select from the following according to the symptoms:

(1) Feels *stiff and painful*, but loosens up with continued motion:

> *Rhus toxicodendron 30 6h*

> [potencies lower than 30 may be much less effective]

(2) Symptoms as in (1), but where there is a strong history of back problems, or where the above remedy fails:

> *Calcarea fluorica 6 6h*

> [potencies higher than 6 may cause temporary aggravation]

(3) Feels *bruised*, but loosens up with continued motion. Particularly useful in the prevention and treatment of *gardeners' backache*, especially in the elderly:

> *Bellis perennis 30 6h*

(4) Feels *bruised*, but feels *worse from continued motion*. Particularly useful to minimize the muscular aches of vigorous sporting activities, not only in the back muscles, but generally. May be used preventatively before sports:

> *Arnica 30 6h*

The severe back

Severe lumbago is usually brought on by lifting a heavy object, such as suitcase, in an incorrect manner. The back should be straight, the knees bent, and the object grasped firmly, with its weight distributed equally to both hands. Failure to do this may result in agonizing consequences. Muscles or ligaments may be severely strained, vertebrae may be displaced, and disks may be slipped. Where the symptoms of lumbago are intense, the remedies mentioned above may well be inadequate. Consider instead:

(1) Violent backache, the slightest movement agonizing, cold sweat, dragging down feeling:

Antimonium tartaricum 6 6h

(2) Should this fail, or be unavailable, consider:

Bryonia 30 6h

Sciatica

The term for pain due to pressure on the sciatic nerve, radiating down the thigh and leg into the foot. The pain may be mild, but is more usually severe. It may be associated with vertebral displacement, slipped disk, or degenerative arthritis of the spine. It is often brought on by incorrect lifting of heavy objects. It may also arise because of immobility whilst travelling. The following remedies should be considered:

(1) In many *left-sided* cases:

Colocynthis 30 2h

(2) In many *right-sided* cases:

Magnesia phosphorica 30 2h

(3) In cases brought on by prolonged immobility whilst travelling, where sitting worsens the problem, and walking bent over improves it:

Ammonium muriaticum 6 2h

(4) Frequently indicated in the elderly:

Arsenicum album 6 6h

Stiff-neck (Torticollis)

This is the term for spasm in the neck muscles, causing severe pain, and the head to be drawn to one side. In adults, it may arise from exposure of the affected side to a cold draught (eg from a car window), but more commonly is caused by displacement of thoracic vertebrae; that is to say, minor dislocations of the vertebral joints *below* the neck. In some cases the pain may radiate into the shoulder, down the arm, mimicking *tennis elbow*, and into the hand. The most frequent causes of thoracic vertebral displacement are: prolonged car journeys, heavy car steering, ball games, sailing, incorrect lifting, and soft beds. The following remedies should be considered:

(1) Stiff-neck from exposure to a draught:

   Aconite 30 4

(2) In many other cases:

   Lachnantes 30 4h

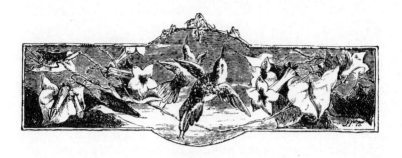

Section 8

FOR WOMEN TRAVELLERS

Whilst covering other topics, this section will be of particular interest with regard to the safety of natural medicines in pregnancy, and during lactation.

PREGNANCY

Immunization

Conventional immunization techniques involving the use of live virus vaccines, or those that are likely to produce a high fever, should be avoided in pregnancy. These include vaccinations against polio (oral vaccine), yellow fever, diphtheria, typhoid, and cholera. Certain antimalarial drugs should not be given. Homoeopathic alternatives, which are perfectly safe in pregnancy, are available, but their statistical efficacy is yet to be established. Please refer to *Section 3*.

Air travel

The major airlines generally allow air travel up to 27 weeks of pregnancy without medical certification, after 28 weeks with medical certification of fitness to travel, but disallow air-travel from 35 weeks (international flights), or 36 weeks (domestic flights). The *optimum* period for travelling, whatever the mode of transport, is 18–24 weeks. Prolonged immobility during a flight, or indeed during any journey, increases the risk of ankle swelling and, more importantly, of serious clots developing in the deep veins of the legs. It is, thus, of the utmost importance that the pregnant woman gets out of her seat occasionally to exercise her legs. Loose clothing should be worn. Pregnant women with the following problems should not fly: anaemia (haemoglobin less than 8.5g/dl), high blood pressure, a history of previous vaginal bleeding, low-lying placenta, and sickle cell trait.

Other forms of travel
Bumpy or rough journeys, including sea voyages, should be avoided in the first 16 and last 4 weeks of pregnancy, and by those with a low-lying placenta, or history of previous vaginal bleeding. *Morning sickness* may be exacerbated by rough seas. Deficiency of *zinc or B vitamins* may render the pregnant woman more prone to the development of *travel-sickness*. Those with sickle cell trait should avoid areas of high altitude.

Anaemia
Air travel, even in pressurised aircraft, or trips to high altitudes should be avoided, if anaemia is present. The main symptoms of anaemia are fatigue, pallor, and breathlessness. Those on *iron medicines* should take adequate amounts of *vitamin C*, either as tablets or as fruit, in order to promote the absorption of iron. Iron medicines should be kept away from children, to whom they may be *highly poisonous*. The requirement for the vitamin *folic acid* is increased in pregnancy, and deficiency may not only contribute to the generation of anaemia, but also render the woman more prone to the development of *tropical sprue* (see the end of this section).

Nutrition and exercise
Maintain adequate nutrition, and avoid excessive exertion (especially in hot climates), dehydration, salt depletion,

alcohol, and tobacco. Severe dehydration encourages miscarriage.

Safe homoeopathic prescriptions

With only the odd exception (which, in any event, is identified in the text), all the homoeopathic remedies mentioned in this manual, when prescribed in the potency range *6c* to *30c* or *12x* to *30x*, are to be considered as safe at any stage of pregnancy, provided that they are stopped immediately if *homoeopathic aggravation* occurs (see *Section 1*). This, however, is a rare event. Whilst such aggravation is *harmless*, if the remedy is discontinued, the administration of several cups of *coffee* will accelerate the reduction of ill-effects.

Medicinal substances to be used with caution

Whilst many medicinal substances, in addition to those described above, are perfectly safe in pregnancy, a considerable number may be harmful. For *internal* use, therefore, you are cautioned not to take any of the medicinal substances listed below without taking proper *professional advice*, preferably from an homoeopathic physician or homoeopathic pharmacist:

Homoeopathic remedies not mentioned in this book.
Homoeopathic remedies bearing potency numbers less than 6, 6c, 6cH, 12x, or D12.
Homoeopathic remedies bearing potency numbers greater than 30, 30c, 30cH, 30x, or D30.
Homoeopathic mother tinctures (bearing the label MT, TM, ø, Tincture of, or Tinctura).
Herbal medicines.
Vitamins.
Minerals.
Orthodox drugs.

Miscarriage (Spontaneous abortion)

If miscarriage threatens, as witnessed by vaginal bleeding in early pregnancy, then go to bed, call a physician (where possible), and take:

(1) *Viburnum opulus 30 6h*
(2) *Arnica 30 4h*

Toxoplasmosis

This is a parasitic disease acquired by eating food contaminated with cat faeces. In the adult it causes a glandular fever-like illness, but, in pregnancy, it may be transmitted to the foetus, causing severe deformity or miscarriage. A principal source of infection is *undercooked meat*, which should be avoided. In Hong Kong, for example, it is not unusual for chicken to be served medium rare! *Unpasteurised milk products and pâtés* should also be avoided, since *Listeria* contamination may lead to miscarriage.

Water sterilization techniques

Water sterilization techniques involving *iodine* (see *Section 10*) are not recommended during pregnancy and whilst breast-feeding.

BREAST-FEEDING (LACTATION)

Nutrition

The maintenance of correct nutrition is of the utmost importance. The consumption of *brewer's yeast and kelp tablets (4 daily of each)* may be found helpful. The same supplements may be used safely in pregnancy. Brewer's yeast occasionally causes indigestion, and kelp occasionally causes some looseness of the bowels. Severe exertion in hot climates, in that it may induce dehydration and salt depletion, is to be avoided. Alcohol should not be taken.

Safety of medicines

The rules regarding the safety of medicinal substances, given above, apply equally during lactation. There are, however, two additional points relevant to the latter:

(a) The activity of most homoeopathic remedies does pass into the breast milk. It is, thus, possible to treat a sickly infant by dosing the mother with the remedy indicated for the child. On the other hand, only *seldom* will the baby be affected by a remedy clearly indicated for the treatment of the mother. It is not, therefore, necessary to abandon breast-feeding for the purpose of treating the mother with homoeopathic remedies. In such rare instances where the baby is adversely affected by homoeopathic activity in the breast milk, these disturbances are generally of a minor nature (eg looseness of the motions, excessive crying, minor skin rash). Should the baby be disturbed in any way during treatment of the mother, then it would be wise to abandon the remedy in favour of an alternative, even though another cause for the child's distress would be more likely, and should, indeed, be sought.

(b) *Rarely*, homoeopathic remedies given for some other purpose may modify the production of breast milk; a matter which may be good or bad. The remedies *Pulsatilla* and *Urtica urens* are particular culprits in this respect, when taken internally. They should not be taken, therefore, during lactation, unless the patient is prepared for, or indeed desires, some change in the flow of breast milk (see below).

Advantages of breast-feeding
The maintenance of the sterility of bottles, and the availability of hygienic milk supplies may both be problematical in remote or developing areas, especially where the climate is hot. Breast-feeding is the sensible alternative, especially as it has more general advantages for both mother and infant. It may, however, be jeopardised by the development of *breast abscess*, or *cracked nipples*. In some, the milk supply simply becomes *insufficient*. For these matters, homoeopathic remedies may be taken to great effect.

Breast abscess
This is characterized by severe pain, swelling, hardness, and heat in a segment of the lactating breast, and is due to infection. Advanced cases require the services of a medical practitioner, and incision and drainage may be necessary. Early treatment is, thus, advisable. Consider:

(1) *Phytolacca 30 6h*
(2) *Bryonia 30 6h*

51

Cracked or sore nipples

(1) *Externally*, sparingly apply the following cream:

Cremor Calendulae 5% 3h

(2) Additionally, take the following remedy by mouth:

Castor equi 6 6h

Insufficient milk

Dehydration is one possible cause, and this should be corrected by additional fluid intake. Where this is not the case, lactation may be promoted by:

(1) *Urtica urens 6 6h*
(2) *Pulsatilla 6 12h*

Abandoning lactation (Weaning)

Taking the child from the breast, when deemed appropriate, may result in engorgement and discomfort. This may be prevented by taking:

Lac caninum 200 12h (6 doses only)

SOME IMPORTANT INFECTIONS

Thrush

Hot climates, dehydration, poor hygiene, nylon underwear, and tight jeans increase the predisposition to vaginal yeast infections. Nutritionally, a high intake of sugars, other than in the form of fresh fruit, may also be contributory. Thrush is a common complication of antibiotic therapies. It is characterized by a thick, white, itchy, non-offensive discharge, with reddening of the vulva. It may be communicated to an infant, with the development of thick white patches in the mouth, which cannot be scraped off easily. What appears to be a severe nappy (diaper) rash may be associated. Oral thrush is also commonly seen in adults taking antibiotics, where it usually presents as soreness, with white spots on a reddened background. For both vaginal and oral thrush, sugar intake should be drastically reduced, and the following remedy considered:

Borax 30 6h

Intertrigo (Inflammation of skin folds)
Increased sweating, and poor hygiene in hot climates may lead to the development of soggy, weeping inflammation in skin-fold areas. It may occur beneath the breasts, especially if large and pendulous, between the buttocks, and behind the ears. Fungal infection is often present. In addition to regular washing, consider the treatment suggested in *Section 16*.

Acute cystitis (Bladder infection)
Far more common in women than men, hot climates, dehydration, and poor hygiene contribute to the development of cystitis. The symptoms include burning or stinging on passing water, frequent desire to pass water, and, in some cases, the appearance of blood in the urine. The presence of a high temperature, and severe pain on tapping the back in the kidney area will indicate a more severe infection of the urinary system, and the services of a physician should be sought. Most cases, however, are less serious, and the following combined regime may be found helpful:

(1) Drink plenty of clean water.
(2) Avoid all acid (sharp) fruits.
(3) Avoid alcoholic drinks.
(4) Take *barley* in any form (eg barley water, boiled barley, barley soup), if available, several times daily.
(5) Take:

Triticum repens ø 10 drops 3h

(6) Additionally, take:
(a) *Cantharis 30 6h*, or
(b) *Staphysagria 6 6h*

In order to *prevent* cystitis in those predisposed to it, the following measures are useful:

(1) Avoid white wines, cider, and excesses of alcohol in general.

(2) Avoid acid (sharp) fruits, and their juices, such as orange and grapefruit.

(3) Avoid dehydration, especially when exercising.

(4) Shower at least once daily, and especially after intercourse.

(5) Wear cotton underwear.

(6) *Stigmata maidis (Cornsilk) tea, one cup daily*, should be taken. It is prepared as follows:

Infuse 1 level teaspoon of dried cornsilk in 1 cup of boiling water for 10 minutes. Strain and drink.

This same herbal tea may also be used with some effect in the *treatment* of acute cystitis, where *Triticum repens* ø is not available (see above). Here the dose would be *1 cup 6h*.

FOLIC ACID SUPPLEMENTATION

Supplementary *folic acid*, under medical guidance, should be considered for all women who are pregnant, or who are taking female hormones, including the contraceptive pill, when visiting the following areas: India, Sri Lanka, the Himalayas, South-East Asia, the Far East, northern Australia, South and Central America. For further details concerning this matter, see *Tropical sprue (Section 10)*.

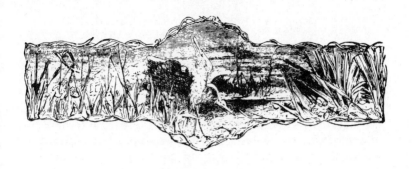

Section 9

TOURISTS' CONSTIPATION

Whilst the avoidance of travellers' diarrhoea often preoccupies the tourist, the occurrence of constipation may be an almost equally unpleasant, if less inconvenient, state. Regrettably, it is extremely *common*. Constipation may be defined as the *delayed or difficult passage of motions*. The abdomen becomes bloated and uncomfortable, the appetite impaired, the sense of motivation depressed, the energy depleted, and haemorrhoids (piles) are aggravated. Its causes are several:

Constrictive clothing
The wearing of clothing that constricts the abdomen, such as tight belts and corsetry, impairs the action of the intestine. Such an effect will be enhanced by the expansion of intestinal gas on ascent during air travel, fluid retention before periods or in response to hot climates, increase in abdominal fat from overeating, the consumption of carbonated drinks, the consumption of fermentable foods (eg beans, cabbage), and prolonged immobility in the seated position. It is, therefore,

55

advisable to wear *loose clothing* for all but the shortest journeys.

Dehydration

Depletion of the water reserves of the body leads to hardening of the faeces. Delays at airports with insufficient refreshment, long car journeys with infrequent stops, low aircraft humidity, increased exercise, and hot climates are frequently contributory. *Alcohol*, by increasing the excretion of water via the kidneys, is also a major factor. *Most travellers do not sufficiently maintain their state of hydration even in the early stages of a vacation.*

Change of diet

A certain amount of dietary *vegetable fibre* is necessary for normal function of the gut. Any significant *deviation* from the traveller's normal intake, either in terms of quantity, type, or distribution between meals, will lead to problems. The typical *British diet*, for example, provides a good intake of bran fibre at breakfast time in the form of cereal, and a significant quantity of vegetable fibre in the main meal of the day. To be told that most of those most excellent vegetables to be found in Roman markets go mainly to make minestrone soup is but little consolation to the British intestine. The *Continental diet* with which one is normally presented provides fibre largely in the form of salad and fruit. This deviation from the norm is often the cause of constipation (moreover, as will be discussed in *Section 10*, salad and fruit in hot countries, when incorrectly prepared, may be a source of intestinal infection, and travellers' diarrhoea). Conversely, travellers to the United Kingdom, may also become constipated when subjected to a diminished intake of salad and fruit. It is what you are used to that counts. British travellers are advised to take their own supply of *bran cereal* on any trips abroad, a measure which will be, to some degree, a remedy for the problem. A modicum of *self-catering* is better than total reliance on restaurant fare.

Biological clock disturbance

Rapid transportation across time-zones via modern air travel, or any prolonged journey with disturbance of the normal sleeping pattern may result in constipation. For a fuller discussion of this phenomenon and its homoeopathic amelioration, please see *Jet-lag (Section 5)*.

Suppression of 'call to stool'
The so-called *call to stool* is that feeling in the abdomen or rectal area that informs us of the need to pass motions. Should it be ignored for more than a few minutes, it will pass, and constipation will frequently ensue. Such suppression of the desire to defaecate may be due to various factors, including: lack of availability of toilets, linguistic barriers to finding such, reluctance to defaecate in public toilets, reluctance to defaecate in shared holiday accommodation, and the reluctance to use insanitary toilets (which latter may be a wise decision!). Provided there is no infective risk to health, pass motions where you can, when Nature determines such is appropriate.

The treatment of constipation
Having discussed the causes and prevention of constipation, it now remains to formulate its treatment, should it occur, despite attempts otherwise:

Increase your consumption of clean water.

Take bran cereals each morning.

Increase your consumption of cooked vegetable dishes, especially modestly spiced ones (note that raw vegetables may be a source of intestinal infection in hot countries, if inadequately cleaned).

Reduce your intake of cooked meats.

Avoid alcoholic drinks.

Wear loose clothing, so as not to constrict the abdomen.

Additionally, the use of homoeopathic remedies should be considered, according to the *individualised symptoms*:

(1) Obstinate constipation, with *no desire whatsoever to pass motions*:

    Opium 6 6h

(2) Constipation, with *frequent ineffectual urging*:

Nux vomica 6 6h

(3) Constipation, with aggravation of *piles* (*haemor-rhoids*), which are painful and may bleed:

Hydrastis 6 6h

Should these remedies fail, or be unavailable, consider the following proprietary preparations, obtainable from pharmacies:

(1) *Syrupus Ficorum (BPC 1934) 7½ ml (1½ standard teaspoons) by mouth each night before retiring.* The dose should be reduced for children (see *Section 2*). For those who wish to prepare it themselves, the instructions are as follows: *Add 40g of finely chopped figs to 100ml of boiling water. Prepare a decoction by simmering gently for 1 hour. Strain, express, and wash pulp with hot water to produce 100ml. Simmer gently again to reduce volume to 50ml. Dissolve 67½g of sugar (cane or beet) in the warm liquid, and adjust to 100ml with clean water.*

(2) *Syrupus Ficorum Compositus (BPC) 7½ml (1½ standard teaspoons) by mouth each night before retiring.* Remember again to reduce the dose for children. This preparation is stronger in action than the above, in that it contains extracts of *Ficus (fig), Rheum (rhubarb), Cascara, Senna, Coriandrum (coriander), and Cardamomi fructus (cardamom seed).*

(3) *Glycerin suppository, one inserted into the rectum each night before retiring.* Different sizes for adults and children are available.

Chronic amoebic dysentery

This disease is associated with alternating bouts of constipation and diarrhoea. The treatment of this condition is discussed in Section 10.

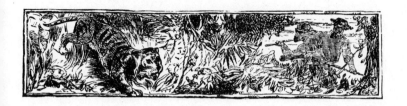

Section 10

TRAVELLERS' DIARRHOEA

Diarrhoea may be defined as *the passage of unformed stools*. Whilst some cases of travellers' diarrhoea may be due to a change in diet, such as eating excessively spicy dishes, or nervous upsets, the majority are due to the ingestion of food or drink contaminated with microorganisms or their toxic products. Commoner in visitors to hot or developing countries, it has been estimated that approximately 40% of international travellers are affected by this unpleasant condition, with 30% of those so afflicted being confined to bed. *Travellers' diarrhoea* is not, however, a single disorder, but rather a *group of disorders* caused by different microorganisms and their toxins, producing different effects, but all characterized by a dominant symptom of *diarrhoea*. Other symptoms may include the passage of blood, nausea, vomiting, or fever. The careful management of food and water hygiene is of paramount importance in its prevention.

Food hygiene
Hands should be washed, and carefully dried, before either preparing or eating food. Cutlery and plates should be free

59

of food residues, and dry. *Meat* should be well-cooked (undercooked meat may also be a source of other diseases, such as toxoplasmosis, and worm infestations). Similarly, *fish* should be well-cooked; eat it raw at your own peril! Cooked foods should be served immediately, or covered, to protect them from microorganisms, including those carried by flies, and refrigerated straight away. Good old-fashioned sticky fly-papers, or fly-killing lamps do much to reduce the risk of contamination from flies, both methods being essentially non-toxic, and, in this sense, preferable to chemical insecticides in food preparation areas. Beware of reheated *soups*! Raw foods, such as *salad vegetables*, should be washed thoroughly in clean water. This is all the more important in areas where human faeces are used as fertilizer, a practice widespread in tropical countries. In all countries where the microbiological purity of the water cannot be guaranteed, when eating out, the consumption of salads and raw vegetables should be avoided. Similarly, *fruit* should preferably be washed in clean water, and then peeled before being eaten. Even if not washed, it should be peeled. However, beware of Egyptian melons injected with contaminated water in order to increase their weight. Shake them before purchase. If the slopping sound of water is heard, do not buy them. *Rice* is yet another problem, if not consumed fairly soon after cooking, or inadequately reheated. A bacterium called *Bacillus cereus* is a common contaminant of rice (even in developed Western countries), and produces a toxin. If the toxin is produced within the rice, vomiting some 1–5 hours after consumption is a dominant feature. Alternatively, consumption of these organisms may result in the toxin being generated within the intestine, with severe diarrhoea occurring some 8–16 hours after eating. Freshly cooked rice is generally safe. *Unpasteurised milk and milk products* should be avoided (which may also be a source of tuberculosis, brucellosis, and listeriosis). *Shellfish* are a common cause of food-related illness, since they are often gathered in waters contaminated with human faecal material, and should definitely be avoided in hot weather. Neither would I recommend *pâtés* in hot climates. As a general rule, when eating out in countries of doubtful hygienic standard, avoid the preprepared foods to be found on market stalls, and avoid 'cheap' restaurants.

Water hygiene

Clean water should be used for both drinking, and tooth-cleaning. The hazards of cleaning raw foods with dirty water have been mentioned above. Utensils, crockery, cutlery, and hands ideally should also be washed in pure water, and thoroughly dried. Where the purity of water cannot be guaranteed, the average traveller is advised to use *bottled water*, where possible, and drinks containing *ice* should be avoided. With regard to bottled water, ensure that the factory seal is intact, for it is not unknown for bottles to be refilled with doubtful water by the unscrupulous. For extra security, purchase carbonated water, which is less likely to be bogus. The strength of alcohol in alcoholic beverages is insufficient to kill many noxious organisms. *Swimming* in contaminated waters is another source of infection, often ignored.

Where bottled water is unavailable, it is possible, however, to purify that locally available. *Boiling vigorously for 5 minutes* is the most effective method of sterilization, in that it destroys all relevant organisms. After boiling, the vessel should be covered, and the water allowed to cool for several hours before drinking, a measure which will significantly improve its 'flat' taste. *Water filtration techniques* are less satisfactory than the former method, and should be regarded as an initial preparation of the water prior to using *chemical sterilization methods*. Indeed, the removal of organic material by filtration prior to chemical sterilization vastly improves its efficacy. Both *chlorine and iodine* have been used, with reasonable safety. Commercially prepared sterilization tablets based on either element are available, but chlorine is less effective than iodine in destroying the cysts of amoebic dysentery organisms. Iodine is, therefore, generally more useful. A simple way of utilising this element is to obtain from your pharmacist *Tincture of Iodine 2%*, and add 4 drops of this tincture to each litre of filtered water, allowing it to stand at least 20 minutes, but preferably 3 hours, before use. Stronger tinctures of iodine are available (eg 10%), but the amount used for sterilization purposes must be proportionately reduced. *Do not use iodine during pregnancy or lactation*.

Homoeopathic prevention

Homoeopathic remedies may be taken to augment those sensible methods of avoidance given above. The use of *Shigella co. nosode* has been mentioned in *Section 3*. However, a more generally useful technique is to take the following remedy on a regular basis throughout the trip:

> *Crataegus ø 5 drops 6h*

This remedy encourages the normal gut organisms, and discourages invading bacteria. It appears that it does not act on the wall of the gut itself, and does not cause constipation. Its side-effects are rare and minor, but the dose should, of course, be reduced for children (see *Section 2*).

Treatment of travellers' diarrhoea

The most important single aspect of therapy in all cases is the *maintenance of adequate fluid intake*. Rehydration sachets, containing glucose and minerals, may be purchased at most pharmacies, and these are added to clean water according to the manufacturers instructions. So important is it to prevent dehydration, especially in infants, it has been said that even water of doubtful purity is better than none. Where rehydration sachets are unavailable, you may make your own rehydration fluids according to a variety of formulae:

(1) *Dissolve 16 level teaspoons of any sugar (including honey), plus 1 level teaspoon of common salt in 2 litres of clean water. This is quick to prepare.*

(2) *Dissolve 25 level teaspoons of rice powder by boiling in a little water. Top up to 2 litres with clean water. Add 1 level teaspoon of salt. This formula, though more difficult to prepare, is better than the above in producing rapid rehydration.*

(3) *Either of the above formulae will be improved by the addition of bicarbonate of soda (sodium bicarbonate). Instead of adding 1 level teaspoon of salt to every 2 litres of liquid, add ½ level teaspoon of salt plus ½ level teaspoon of*

bicarbonate of soda to that amount of liquid. This helps correct the state of bodily acidity (acidosis) that tends to arise as a result of diarrhoeal illness.

Rehydration fluids are best given little and often; initially, sips should be encouraged every 10 or 15 minutes. This is generally successful, but occasionally severe vomiting hampers the treatment. Infants are notorious for not keeping anything down, and a good trick is to feed them on half-set jelly (known as *jello* in North America), which is peculiarly well-tolerated. Many a disaster has been averted with this therapeutic device. Breast-feeding should be continued, even when the diarrhoea is severe, alternating feeds at the breast with the administration of rehydration fluids by bottle, spoon, or dropper. *Severe dehydration* is a medical emergency, especially in infants, and medical assistance should be sought. You must, therefore, be aware of its symptoms. These include: dry tongue, sunken eyes, scanty and dark urine, and a 'doughy' feel to the skin (this latter being due to loss of elasticity – if you pinch the skin of the abdomen between thumb and forefinger, you will notice that it takes several seconds to go flat).

Once the patient is on the road to recovery, normal food, having been denied in favour of rehydration fluids, must be reintroduced. The diet should be low in fat, fibre, and acidity. Potato soup is particularly suitable. Avoid greens, beans, and whole-grain products. Boiled white rice, flavoured with soya sauce, and accompanied by steamed fish is an acceptable meal. Where the feeding of babies has been abandoned in favour of oral rehydration, early refeeding is considered important, but may result in return of the diarrhoea. Results would appear, however, to be more satisfactory if a low-fat, low-lactose feed (such as HN25, Milupa) is used for several days.

Orthodox antidiarrheal drugs, such as codeine phosphate and certain opiate derivatives, are often taken by travellers to reduce the severity of symptoms. Their use, however, cannot be encouraged, in that they may produce cramps, or *prolong* the length of the illness, whilst being potentially hazardous in cases of bloody diarrhoea (dysentery) and for children below 4 years of age. Whereas it has been stated that the primary treatment of travellers' diarrhoea is rehydration, there is, nevertheless, a strong case for using natural, especially homoeopathic, medicines as an adjunct, in order to reduce the severity of symptoms, to *shorten* the length of the illness, and to promote the expulsion of the offending microorganisms. Where vomiting is present, the fact that potentized homoeopathic remedies (those bearing a potency number) are rapidly absorbed via the lining of the mouth is a considerable advantage. For these cases, it is better to crush the pilule, tablet or coarse granules to a fine powder for ease of administration. Alternatively, the patient may be instructed to crush the same between his teeth. Otherwise, liquid potencies or fine granules may be used. The selection of the appropriate adjunctive treatment will depend on the symptomatic picture of the illness, which, to some degree, is dependent upon the nature of the causative organism.

When nursing people with diarrhoea, the stools must be disposed of well away from water supplies and food, and scrupulous personal hygiene must be maintained to prevent the spread of the disease to yourself and others.

Classification of travellers' diarrhoea
From the clinical and therapeutic point of view, travellers' diarrhoea may be classified in accordance with the following main headings:

(1) Common watery diarrhoea:
    (a) Short-lasting (the commonest type of travellers' diarrhoea)
    (b) Persistent (*giardiasis*)
(2) *Tropical sprue*
(3) Bloody diarrhoea (*Dysentery*):
    (a) *Bacillary dysentery* (usually short-lasting)
    (b) *Amoebic dysentery* (persistent)
(4) *Cholera*

Short-lasting watery diarrhoea
This is by far the commonest type of travellers' diarrhoea. It is known affectionately by various names, such as *Turista*,

Delhi Belly, Tutenkhamen's Curse, and Montezuma's Revenge. It is caused by a variety of organisms, including: the bacteria, enterotoxigenic *Escherichia coli* (ETEC), *Salmonellae, Vibrio parahaemolyticus*, and *Aeromonas hydrophilia*; Rotaviruses; and the protozoon *Cryptosporidium*. The incubation period is generally no longer than 4 days, and often shorter. There is a sudden onset of profuse watery diarrhoea, and abdominal cramps. Fever may or may not be present. Without medication, it usually resolves in 1–5 days, but rarely may continue for 14 days. The following prescriptions should be considered:

(1) The *key* remedy in many cases, which should be continued until the stools return to a normal consistency:

> *Arsenicum album 6 2h*
>
> [here, the optimum potency range for this remedy is 6 to 12; potencies higher than 12 may be *less* effective in treating diarrhoea]

(2) In severe cases, where no improvement has been seen after 24 hours treatment with the above, consider the following daily rotation of remedies, repeating the sequence until the stools return to a normal consistency:

> DAY 1: *Cinchona officinalis 30 6h*
> DAY 2: *Arsenicum album 6 6h*
> DAY 3: *Podophyllum 6 6h*

(3) In conjunction with either prescriptions (1) or (2) given above, the following mixture may be given to fortify the effect:

> *Zingiber ø 5ml +*
> *Crataegus ø 5ml*
> *10 drops in 2 teaspoons of clean water 6h*
>
> [alternatively, you may give simultaneously 5 drops of each mother tincture, if available separately]

Remember to reduce the dose for children (see *Section 2*).

(4) In addition to any of the above, for *severe griping pains*:

> *Colocynthis 30 2h as necessary*

(5) In conjunction with the homoeopathic remedies given above, the provision of *folic acid* supplementation may be indicated, if the bout of diarrhoea arises from a visit to certain countries. For a fuller discussion of this point, see below, under *Tropical sprue*.

(6) If, after 7 days of treatment with the above, no significant improvement in the diarrhoea has occurred, proceed to prescribing notes (10) to (14) given below, under the subsection *Persistent watery diarrhoea*.

(7) Once the diarrhoea has abated, recovery is often hastened by giving the following remedy for several days to a week. It should be continued for 48 hours after apparent total recovery, in order to prevent relapse:

> *Cinchona officinalis 30 6h*

(8) In conjunction with prescription (7) given above, the following may be given to fortify its effect:

> *Crataegus ø 5 drops 6h*

(9) In the absence of appropriate homoeopathic remedies, the spice *Nutmeg (Nux moschata)* has been used to control severe cases of travellers' diarrhoea. A pinch of the finely ground spice may be given directly on the tongue *6h*. However, Nutmeg is *toxic* when taken in larger doses, and it should not be given, without taking proper advice, to small children, epileptics, or pregnant women.

Some diagnostic pitfalls

(i) In the case of a child with watery diarrhoea and fever, it may be due to almost any infection: acute middle-ear infection, tonsillitis, chest infection, urinary infection, and so on. General examination of the child, preferably by a medical professional, is of the utmost importance. Should such an infection be found, then homoeopathic treatment must be instituted to cover this problem. The homoeopathic measures given above may be inadequate. The treatment of some of these problems is discussed in Section 18.

(ii) Malaria (especially the P. falciparum type) may present with the symptoms of watery diarrhoea and fever. Malaria is discussed in Section 20. The therapeutic measures given above will be inadequate.

(iii) Mild cases of shigellosis (see below) may present with fever, watery diarrhoea, but without blood in the stools. Whilst the treatment suggested above will suffice, the recognition of this possibility is of some importance, since the patient, having apparently made a full recovery, may continue to harbour Shigella bacteria for several months, thus constituting a health hazard to others.

(iv) Mild cases of cholera (see below) may present as a brief, self-limiting, watery diarrhoea, with no fever. This may well respond to the above measures, but the patient may become a symptomless carrier of the disease for about 10 days after the illness, and sometimes longer. During a cholera outbreak, even mild cases of watery diarrhoea should be regarded with suspicion.

(v) Diarrhoea may occur as a result of typhoid, for which the treatment is quite different (see Section 23).

(vi) Mild episodes of watery diarrhoea may be associated with psychological upsets, or gastronomic overindulgence. These should be treated in accordance with the principles given in Sections 4 and 11 of this manual.

(vii) Watery diarrhoea may result from ciguatoxic fish poisoning (see Section 11).

Persistent watery diarrhoea (Giardiasis)

Even without medicinal treatment, most cases of watery diarrhoea in travellers recover within 14 days. Watery diarrhoea persisting for more than 14 days frequently implies the presence within the intestine of the protozoan parasite *Giardia lamblia* (hence, the term *giardiasis*). In many instances, the initial phase of watery diarrhoea gives way to the passage of bulky, extremely offensive, fatty, pale stools, a condition that may remain with the patient for weeks, months, or even years. This results from the destruction of the finger-like projections of the lining of the gut, termed *villi*, which are responsible for the absorption of food. Thus, deficiency states may arise as a result of Giardia lamblia infection. The patient may, for example, present several months after a vacation with symptoms resembling *irritable bowel syndrome*, loss of weight, and, occasionally, loss of hair as a result of chronic zinc deficiency. Less than 10% of cases are so affected. Even without treatment, the majority of cases will resolve spontaneously within 3 months.

Identification of the cysts of the parasite within a stool specimen is theoretically possible, but, in practice, may be extremely difficult. From the clinical point of view, infection with this organism is usually inferred from the history. Giardiasis is extremely common in tropical countries, but may also be contracted in other parts, such as Russia and the USA. Since the incubation period is approximately 7 to 21 days, the illness may not appear until the traveller has returned home.

Since, in its initial phase, Giardia infection is symptomatically similar to *short-lasting watery diarrhoea*, homoeopathic treatment at this stage may follow similar lines (see above). However, should these measures fail, other homoeopathic treatment will be indicated:

(10) In many cases of watery diarrhoea, where prescriptions (1)-(5), described above, have been given for 7 days without significant improvement:

Cinchona officinalis 30 6h

(11) If the above remedy should fail:

Oleander 6 6h

(12) Either of the above two remedies should also be considered for the *initial treatment* of cases presenting at the later bulky, pale stool stage of the disease. Resistant cases may respond to either *Pulsatilla* or *Sulphur*, as documented below with regard to *tropical sprue*.

(13) In cases of suspected giardiasis, in addition to the appropriate homoeopathic remedies, the following should be taken:
   (a) *Garlic (Allium sativum)*, several raw fresh cloves daily, or in the form of garlic capsules or tablets, available from pharmacies and health-food stores.
   (b) Non-oily nutritional supplements, especially *vitamin B complex* and *zinc* (adult dose: *30mg elemental zinc daily*). *Vitamin B12 malabsorption* is present in over 50% of cases, and should be

supplied by injection, or as large doses by mouth (adult dose: *500mcg daily*). Folic acid, calcium, and iron supplements are not generally required.

(14) The services of a medical practitioner should be sought in all cases of persistent diarrhoea which have not responded to the suggested treatment.

Some additional points

(i) Some cases of persistent watery diarrhoea are due to secondary disaccharidase deficiency; that is to say, an acquired inability to digest certain sugars, especially lactose (milk sugar). Such cases may be resistant to the treatment suggested above, but will respond to a milk-free diet. Homoeopathic tablets and powders usually contain lactose, and should not be prescribed. However, homoeopathic pilules, coarse granules, and fine granules are generally made from sucrose, and should, therefore, present no problem in the case of lactose intolerance. Use liquid potencies if in doubt. Milk may generally be reintroduced after several months.

(ii) Damage to the wall of the small intestine by Escherichia coli bacteria may, especially in children, produce a picture similar to that described for giardiasis. The treatment, moreover, is along similar lines to those given above. Giardia, of course, will be undetectable in stool specimens.

Tropical sprue

This mysterious disorder has certain clinical and pathological features in common with giardiasis (see above), with which, in its early stages, it may be confused. It is generally held that this disorder is caused by the colonization of the upper intestine by coliform bacteria in individuals exhibiting deficiency states (especially folic acid, and, secondarily, iron). Travellers are not exempt! As with some cases of giardiasis, destruction of the intestinal *villi* (see above) occurs, giving rise, however, to a considerably greater state of malabsorption, and serious multiple deficiencies. Tropical sprue is endemic in India, Sri Lanka, the Himalayas, South-East Asia, the Far East, northern Australia, and both South and Central America. Epidemics of sprue still occur in India. In eastern India, the epidemic sprue season coincides, not surprisingly, with the fly season; March to September, with a maximum incidence in June.

Typically, the disease begins with explosive and watery

diarrhoea, abdominal cramps, and vomiting. At this stage it resembles other more common varieties of travellers' diarrhoea. Gradually, the stools change to those typical of a malabsorption state. They become pale, fatty, porridge-like, and highly offensive (rather like the later stages of giardiasis), and are exacerbated by the consumption of fats. The diarrhoea usually occurs at night or in the morning, preceded by abdominal colic and a feeling of great urgency, which symptoms are immediately relieved by its passage. Extreme fatigue is experienced, and weight may be lost at the rate of approximately 7kg per month. Appetite may be absent, or present, yet with an inability to consume more than a few morsels of food. After about 6 weeks, ulcers often appear in the mouth, following which both the tongue and the lining of the mouth become painfully red and angry. Difficulty in swallowing, and vomiting may occur. After about 4 months, anaemia becomes apparent. The skin becomes rough, dry, and pigmented. The patient is obviously profoundly ill. This is the picture of classical tropical sprue. The severity of this disorder readily distinguishes it from the latter stages of giardiasis. However, cases with much milder symptoms are now becoming more common, especially in travellers, and may cause some diagnostic confusion (often there is no inflammation of the tongue, and anaemia is not present). The matter of differentiation is of considerable importance, in that an established case of tropical sprue will require a significantly different treatment.

In the initial watery diarrhoea phase, homoeopathic treatment may be given along the lines suggested previously for common watery diarrhoea, from which, at this stage, it will be clinically indistinguishable. Such treatment, however, may well fail unless *folic acid* (a B vitamin) is given simultaneously (by injection, or orally; adult dose: *15mg daily*). There is a strong case, therefore, for the routine administration of folic acid to all cases of watery diarrhoea occurring in those countries in which tropical sprue is endemic (see above). Pregnant women are particularly prone to folic acid deficiency, and should take it routinely (after the first trimester) when visiting these areas (*0.5mg daily*). During the first trimester, *dried brewer's yeast tablets, three twice daily after food*, will provide a safe and useful quantity of folic acid (100g of dried brewer's yeast contains 2.4mg of folic acid). *Iron* deficiency in such ladies should also be corrected, by the provision of iron supplements and *vitamin C* (after the first trimester). Other groups prone to folic acid deficiency, and, therefore, similarly at risk, include: women taking the contraceptive pill, or other forms of female hormone therapy; the elderly; those who drink alcohol regularly (even if they are not alcoholics as such); and those taking certain drugs, especially aspirin, cholestyramine, phenytoin, primidone, pyrimethamine (commonly used as a malarial preventative), and triamterene. Such groups should also take oral folic acid as a preventative (adult dose: *0.5mg daily*), but those taking the drug phenytoin must consult their physicians, since extra folic acid may neutralize its effect.

Established cases of tropical sprue, when the stools have changed to the offensive, porridge-like stage, will require *both* nutritional and homoeopathic therapy along the following lines:

(1) *All cases should be given folic acid*! In cases of tropical sprue of less than one year's duration, dramatic improvement occurs. Appetite returns, the weight increases, the mouth returns to normal, and, in the absence of iron deficiency, the state of anaemia remits. The diarrhoea, though suffering an initial exacerbation, subsequently improves. This is quite different from giardiasis, which is not improved by folic acid supplementation (see above). Folic acid may be given either by injection, or orally (adult dose: *10–20mg daily, depending upon the severity of the case*). However, since severe neurological damage may arise when folic acid is given in the face of untreated vitamin B12 deficiency, another deficiency state common in tropical sprue, it is prudent to give *vitamin B12* supplementation concurrently. This may be given by injection, or orally in large doses (*500mcg daily*). In cases where pallor and fatigue persist, despite these remedial measures, iron deficiency may be suspected, especially in females, and iron supplementation plus vitamin C, to encourage its absorption, should

be given (such as *ferrous fumarate 200mg three times daily, plus vitamin C 200mg three times daily, given together after food*). Whilst the initial improvement is dramatic, relapses will frequently occur if medicinal methods are not also applied to the case. A combined nutritional and homoeopathic treatment is, therefore, of the utmost importance. The homoeopathic therapy now follows.

(2) A prescription frequently indicated, which should be continued for many months:

Pulsatilla 6 12h

[avoid using potencies higher than 12]

(3) Alternatively, where the above remedy fails to prevent relapse, especially in cases where *morning diarrhoea* is present, consider the following, which should be used for many months:

Sulphur 6 12h

[avoid using potencies higher than 9]

(4) In conjunction with the above, in order to fortify the effect, give:

Crataegus ø 5 drops 6h

[reduce the dose for children]

(5) *Repatriation* of the traveller to a *temperate climate* of origin, provided that the disease is of less than one year's duration, often produces spontaneous improvement. Such people should not be allowed to return to a hot climate without the provision of *folic acid* (adult dose: *5mg daily*). Patients who are so repatriated after the disease has been present for one year, may suffer frequent relapses, which, paradoxically, often occur during the winter and spring, rather than the summer. Such cases require specialist homoeopathic treatment, and are best referred to the homoeopathic physician.

Some diagnostic pitfalls

Giardiasis and tropical sprue are not the only causes of persistent (chronic) fatty diarrhoea relevant to the traveller. Others, which will require substantially different treatment, include:

(i) Gluten sensitivity (late-onset coeliac disease), which may develop in the tropics. Here, the patient must exclude wheat, barley, and rye from the diet.

(ii) Tuberculosis of the abdominal lymph-glands.

(iii) Abdominal lymphoma (a form of malignancy).

(iv) Chronic pancreatitis (especially in the inhabitants of Africa, Indonesia, and southern India).

(v) Strongyloidiasis, a nematode worm infection (see small-print note to 'Creeping eruption' in Section 16).

(vi) Capillaria philippinensis, a nematode worm infecting the small intestine; acquired by eating raw freshwater fish, and found in the Philippines, Thailand, Egypt, and Iran.

(vii) Alpha chain disease, found particularly in the Eastern Mediterranean, and the Arabian peninsula.

(viii) Pellagra (caused by deficiency of the B vitamin nicotinic acid and other substances).

Persistent diarrhoea with fever and wasting

In the tropics, the association of these three symptoms is strongly indicative of tuberculosis, AIDS, or, where it is known to be endemic, of visceral leishmaniasis (see Section 26).

Bloody diarrhoea (Dysentery)

Diarrhoea with blood occurs much less frequently than watery diarrhoea. It accounts for no more than 15% of the total number of cases of travellers' diarrhoea. Dysentery may occur as a short-lasting illness, caused by bacteria, or as a persistent illness, usually caused by parasitic infection. The most common variety of the former is *bacillary dysentery (shigellosis)*, and of the latter, *amoebic dysentery*. Table 10.1 summarises the salient differences between these two principal diseases, and will help you to make a proper diagnosis. Where there is some difficulty in reaching a diagnosis, remember that *the presence or absence of fever* is a key point in differentiating between the two diseases. A fuller discussion of the dysenteries and their homoeopathic treatment follows this table.

Table 10.1

Bacillary dysentery	Amoebic dysentery
Short-lasting (less than 21 days).	*Persistent* (more than 21 days).
Sudden onset.	Usually develops slowly.
Fever common.	**Fever usually absent.**
Initial vomiting.	No vomiting.
Stools scanty, but frequent.	Stools often copious.
Stools like *red currant jelly, or pink frog-spawn*.	Faeces mixed with blood & mucus.
Stools *odourless*.	Stools *offensive*.
Severe rectal spasms.	Rectal spasms unusual.
Short incubation period.	Long incubation period.
Often epidemic (occurring in outbreaks).	Endemic (ingrained in the community).
Complications: arthritis, eye problems.	Complications: liver & other 'abscesses', perforation of gut, amoebiasis of skin.

Bacillary dysentery (Shigellosis)
This disorder is caused by bacteria of the *Shigella* group. Shigellosis occurs in both temperate and tropical climates, and outbreaks are not unknown even in the United Kingdom. The most severe forms of the disease, however, usually occur in the tropics and East Asia. The peak incidence in hot countries occurs in early summer, whilst in temperate climates, the peak incidence is during the winter. The disease may be transmitted via both food and water. Flies are an important vector. Where bacteriological facilities are available, the organisms are readily recovered, and thus identified, from *fresh* stool mucus (slime). Homoeopathic

preventative measures have been discussed above, and in *Section 3*.

The incubation period is variable, but is generally about 3 days. In severe cases, there is a sudden onset of fever, and abdominal pain (colic). Initially, the stools are loose and frequent, without the presence of mucus (slime) or blood. Blood-stained mucus then appears in the motions. This soon gives way to the frequent passage of bloody mucus, up to 60 times daily. These stools are odourless, contain very little faecal material, and resemble, depending on the amount of blood present, red currant jelly or pink frog-spawn. Colic continues to be severe, and distressing rectal spasms occur, which may last up to 30 minutes after the passage of a motion. Urination is also painful. Fortunately, whilst some vomiting may occur at the onset of the disease, it is not a prominent feature subsequently, thus facilitating oral rehydration. Without medicinal treatment the illness generally resolves within 14–21 days, the blood disappearing, and the stools gradually returning to normal. Occasionally, the illness may enter a persistent phase, with the passage of stools containing blood and mucus for many months.

In mild cases, there is little or no fever, and up to 8 loose motions daily are passed, with or without small amounts of blood and mucus, the illness resolving spontaneously in 2–3 days. The recognition of even mild cases is of some considerable importance, in that, during an outbreak of shigellosis, approximately 10% of patients become carriers of the disease for up to 4 months after their illness, whilst exhibiting no symptoms, thus constituting an infective hazard to others via their faeces.

Complications include: inflammation of the eyes (mild conjunctivitis, or, more rarely, iritis); inflammatory arthritis in the convalescent phase (especially of knees and ankles); haemorrhoids (piles) or prolapse of the rectum (projection through the anus), from straining, especially in the malnourished; perforation of the gut, which is rare.

Oral rehydration is satisfactory in many cases, but some may require intravenous fluids. Additionally, the following homoeopathic treatment may be considered:

(1) In the initial phase, where blood is absent, treatment may begin with the measures suggested for *short-lasting watery diarrhoea* (see above), from which it may be clinically indistinguishable.

(2) Where blood has appeared in the motions, give the following combined treatment, repeating it daily until significant improvement occurs:

> *Ipecacuanha 6 a single dose each morning*
> *Petroleum 30 a single dose each evening*
>
> [if you do not have the recommended potencies, substitute any potency of either remedy in the range 6–30]

(3) Should the above prescription fail, consider:

> *Mercurius corrosivus 6 6h*

(4) In conjunction with either (2) or (3), given above, the following may be given, in order to fortify the effect:

> *Crataegus ø 5 drops 6h*
>
> [reduce the dose for children]

(5) In conjunction with any of the above, where there is severe colic or rectal spasm, add:

> *Colocynthis 30 2h as necessary*

(6) To promote recovery, after the diarrhoea has abated, give plenty of *garlic* and:

> *Cinchona officinalis 30 6h*
>
> [and continue with *Crataegus ø 5 drops 6h* for several weeks]

(7) For persistent cases (lasting more than 21 days), give plenty of *garlic* and consider:

> *Sulphur 6 12h*
>
> [avoid using potencies higher than 9]

(8) For haemorrhoids (piles) or rectal prolapse, following a bout of shigellosis:

Podophyllum 6 12h

(9) For conjunctivitis (mild inflammation and soreness of the eyes):

Euphrasia 6 6h

(10) For iritis (severe pain and redness of eye, with tenderness on pressure, and small pupil), whilst trying to obtain urgent medical advice, give:

Rhus toxicodendron 30 12h

(11) For arthritic complications:

Eupatorium perfoliatum 30 12h

Other causes of acute bloody diarrhoea with fever

Bacterial infection with Campylobacter jejuni (mainly a disease of childhood in developing countries), the Salmonellae, and some strains of Escherichia coli may produce a disease clinically identical to shigellosis. The homoeopathic treatment will be the same as that described for the latter.

Amoebic dysentery

This disorder is caused by the amoebic parasite *Entamoeba histolytica*. This organism is found in temperate climates, such as in Great Britain, northern Europe, and the USA, but is commoner in the tropics and subtropics. In many hot countries, a large percentage of the population are symptomless carriers of this parasite, which is excreted in the stools in the form of spherical microscopic *amoebic cysts*, the ingestion of which may induce disease in others. Amoebic cysts in water are destroyed by boiling, but chlorination is relatively ineffective. It is now apparent that there are many strains of *Entamoeba histolytica*, only a few of which are capable of causing disease (*pathogenic* strains). Sophisticated microbiological tests are required to distinguish the various types. The cyst is the 'resting' phase of the organism, and changes into an active *trophozoite* form after ingestion. Pathogenic trophozoites, depending upon the resistance of the host, may then produce ulceration of the gut lining, giving rise to amoebic dysentery. It is the recovery of these active pathogenic trophozoites from fresh stool specimens that is necessary to confirm the latter diagnosis. The mere presence of the cystic form, in cases of bloody diarrhoea, does not confirm that diagnosis. The term *amoebiasis* denotes the state of harbouring pathogenic forms of Entamoeba histolytica, whether causing active disease or not; it applies, therefore, equally to both sufferers and carriers. In many areas, where sophisticated medical tests are unavailable, the diagnosis of amoebic dysentery will be based solely on the clinical picture, which we shall now consider (see also *Table 10.1*, given above).

The incubation period is from one week to several years, although in most cases it is probably a few months. Its appearance, therefore, may be long after return from abroad. In the well-nourished, previously healthy person (the average traveller), the disease is gradual in onset, and often so mild that the patient is fully ambulant. Loose motions are passed three or four times daily, and these become streaked with blood and mucus (slime). Periods of diarrhoea often alternate with periods of constipation. *There is generally no fever*. Neither is there abdominal colic or rectal spasm.

At the other end of the scale, there is severe amoebic dysentery. This tends to occur in the malnourished, patients taking steroid drugs, pregnant women, children recovering from measles, and people living 'rough', such as soldiers and explorers. The onset may be sudden, with the passage of up to 20 liquid, bloody, offensive stools daily, accompanied by fever, weakness, dehydration, abdominal pain, and rectal spasm. The bowel wall may become so weakened, that careless examination of the abdomen may induce its rupture. Hiccup is considered to be an ominous sign. Without treatment, the mortality rate in such cases may be as high as 70%.

Between these two extremes, many cases exhibiting intermediate symptomatic pictures are seen, and, where possible, all cases should be seen by a physician. In some instances, the disease enters a phase of chronicity (persistence), characterized by alternating phases of diarrhoea and constipation over many months, or even years, interspersed with phases of normality. In such cases, diarrhoea may be provoked by gastronomic indiscretion, exhaustion, or catching a cold.

Possible complications of amoebiasis include:

(a) Perforation of the bowel, which requires surgical intervention. There may be severe abdominal pain, rigidity of the muscles of the abdominal wall, vomiting, or hiccup.

(b) Severe haemorrhage may occur from the erosion of a blood vessel. This requires blood transfusion.

(c) Large masses (termed *amoebomas*) may form in the bowel, and cause obstruction. There will be abdominal distention and constipation. Amoebomas may be confused with malignant tumours, and tuberculosis of the bowel. Medicinal treatment is generally preferable to surgical intervention.

(d) Invasion of the skin by pathogenic amoebae may lead to severe ulceration around the anus, and on the genitalia.

(e) *Amoebic liver 'abscess'*. This is not an abscess in the usual sense of the word, in that it contains no pus. It is due to the liquefaction of an area of the liver by amoebae, and consists of a material that resembles anchovy sauce. In some patients, there is no previous history of dysentery, and it may arise years after an excursion to far-off places. In general, however, it occurs in persons who have resided for a long time in the tropics, and who have a history of dysenteric illness. Its symptoms include: a feeling of fullness in the right side of the abdomen, under the ribs; pain in this area, accentuated by coughing or breathing, which may also be felt in the right shoulder; fever with sweating, which may be periodic (and confused with malaria); loss of appetite and weight; liver tenderness on examination (which is not always present); cough. Special investigations are necessary to confirm the diagnosis, but are seldom available in remote and impoverished areas. There may be confusion diagnostically with fluke abscess, or hydatid cyst (see *Section 27*). Medicinal treatment, rather than surgical, is indicated.

(f) Similar 'abscesses' may occur rarely in the lung, spleen, or brain.

(g) Rectal ulcer. Ulceration in or near the rectum may give rise to rectal spasm and the excessive discharge of mucus, a condition which may be persistent.

We shall now consider the homoeopathic treatment of amoebiasis:

(1) *All cases* (including liver 'abscess', and chronic dysentery) should receive the following remedy, irrespective of the symptomatic picture, and it should be given in conjunction with any other indicated remedies:

Entamoeba histolytica nosode 30 12h

(2) In mild cases of amoebic dysentery, where there is little or no abdominal pain, no rectal spasm, and the patient is ambulant, consider:

Phosphorus 6 12h

(3) In severe cases of amoebic dysentery, with the passage of many bloody motions, abdominal cramps and severe rectal spasms, consider:

Mercurius corrosivus 6 6h

(4) In severe cases of amoebic dysentery, where the patient is collapsed, drowsy and confused, consider:

Baptisia 30 6h

(5) In persistent (chronic) cases of amoebic dysentery, with alternate diarrhoea and constipation persisting for months or years, other remedies will be indicated, the selection of which will depend in part on an assessment of the general characteristics of the patient (*garlic* may also be given regularly):

(a) *Sulphur* is especially indicated in robust, hot individuals, with a tendency to skin disorders. The patient feels generally worse in hot weather, or hot rooms. Diarrhoea occurs largely in the morning, the urge to pass motions driving the patient from bed. During the constipation phase, the stools may be hard, and are passed painfully, with the aggravation of piles, which become sore or itchy. Give:

Sulphur 6 12h

[avoid giving potencies higher than 9]

(b) *Nux vomica* is especially indicated in chilly, irritable, overcritical people, often with sedentary occupations. They often have a history of irregular eating, indigestion, and drowsiness after meals. During the diarrhoea phase, there may be rectal spasm, which is relieved for a short time by the passage of motions, although, in some cases, there may be a background of constant uneasiness in the rectum. In the constipation phase, there is frequent ineffectual urging; expulsion is incomplete and unsatisfactory, with a feeling as if part of the motion has remained unexpelled. Give:

Nux vomica 6 12h

(c) *Sepia* is especially indicated in chilly individuals with a yellowish complexion. Their dislike of cold, and love of heat is often extreme. Their irritability is mainly directed towards close members of the family, and is rarely displayed towards friends. They are generally improved by exercise, and are not sedentary by nature. During the constipation phase, there is little desire or urging for days, and then pain in the rectum, during and long after the passage of motions. There may be a sensation as if there were a ball, weight, or lump in the rectum. Constipation phases tend to be longer than phases of diarrhoea, the latter being aggravated by milky drinks. Give:

Sepia 6 12h

[avoid giving potencies higher than 12]

(6) The treatment of amoebic liver 'abscess' is best left to the physician, where possible. Remedies to be considered include:

(a) Where there is pain in the right side of the upper

abdomen or lower chest, aggravated by coughing or breathing:

Bryonia 6 6h

(b) Where there is loss of appetite, great loss of weight, and the liver is tender:

Lycopodium 6 12h

(c) Where there is pain referred to the right shoulder, or constant pain below the right shoulder blade, especially in cases where there is alternation of diarrhoea and constipation:

Chelidonium majus 6 6h

(d) In conjunction with any of the above prescriptions, or by itself, give:

Carduus marianus ø 5 drops 6h

(7) In cases of rectal ulcer, with excessive mucus discharge and rectal spasm, give:

Aloe 6 6h

Balantidial dysentery (Balantidiasis)

This is a parasitic infection caused by the organism Balantidium coli. It is found in both hot and temperate climates, and may be contracted, in some instances, by contact with pigs. Many cases are symptomless, but some develop a clinical picture almost identical to that of amoebic dysentery, although with a greater likelihood of bowel perforation. Confirmation of balantidiasis may be made by recovering the offending organism from a stool specimen. However, the homoeopathic treatment will be similar to that given above for amoebiasis.

Ulcerative colitis

This non-parasitic disease, common in the West, yet rare in the tropics, may produce a symptomatic picture almost identical to that of amoebic dysentery, from which it may be difficult to differentiate. The rarity of this condition in the tropics may be readily explained in terms of homoeopathic theory. Amoebic dysentery, even in its minor form, is homoeopathic to the disease ulcerative colitis. That is to say, it is of such a similarity that, on the basis of the principle 'like prevents like', it negates the predisposition to the latter disorder. Based upon these interesting observations,

I have, in some cases of ulcerative colitis, demonstrated a significant improvement by the administration of Entamoeba histolytica nosode.

Other causes of persistent bloody diarrhoea
These include the following, for which the treatment will be different from that described above:
(i) Bilharziasis, a blood fluke infection (see Section 21).
(ii) Heavy intestinal fluke (flatworm) infections (mostly in South-East Asia).
(iii) Trichuriasis (with heavy infection); a disease caused by whipworms (see Section 27).
(iv) Cancers of the large bowel.

Cholera (formerly termed 'Asiatic cholera')
This disease is caused by the bacterium *Vibrio cholerae*. It is a disease of poor sanitation and hygiene, and may spread to any part of the World where such conditions prevail. Travellers at particular risk are those who visit India, Bengal, South-East Asia, the Middle East, Africa, eastern Europe, South America, and the western Pacific. In these areas, many people are symptomless carriers of the disease. The matter of immunization has been discussed in *Section 3* of this manual, but an additional method is outlined below.

The disease is contracted by the ingestion of food or water contaminated with cholera organisms, which are excreted in the stools of those with active disease and carriers. Since the organism is readily destroyed by stomach acid, the ingestion of large quantities of water, the taking of antacids, and a past history of peptic ulcer operation are conducive to successful infection. The incubation period may be as short as a few hours, or as long as 7 days, but, most typically, is about 48 hours. There is a sudden onset, with explosive diarrhoea. Once the faecal matter has been expelled, copious stools with the appearance of 'rice-water' are produced in phenomenal quantities, from which the offending bacterium may be readily recovered and identified. The expulsion of this liquid is *painless* and effortless, and up to 20 litres may be lost per day. Vomiting, often projectile, but unaccompanied by nausea, is characteristic, occurring in 80% of cases, and significantly interferes with oral rehydration. Severe muscular cramps develop, beginning in the legs, and then becoming more generalised. Fever is unusual, except in children, and the temperature may become subnormal. Without rehydration, the patient becomes exceedingly thirsty, with obvious signs of dehydration, including sunken eyes, wrinkled skin, and diminished urinary output. The breath smells of acetone. Kidney failure and shock follow. The lips become blue, the extremities cold, and an increasing lethargy gives way to terminal coma, and, finally, death. This is the picture of severe cholera. Fortunately, the majority of individuals who become infected with the cholera organism either remain symptomless, or experience only a mild diarrhoeal illness. Less than one seventh of infected individuals develop the symptoms of severe cholera. After infection, with or without symptoms, most individuals will be host to the organism for about 10 days further, and will thus be capable of transmitting the disease to others. Some individuals, however, exhibit a persistent carrier state, and constitute an even greater hazard.

The principal cause of death in severe cholera is depletion of water and minerals. Provided that these are supplied in adequate quantities, complete recovery will ensue. Nursing the patient on a 'cholera cot', a stretcher with a hole cut in the middle, through which the stools are collected in a bucket below, facilitates the measurement of lost fluid, and thus the calculation of that required for rehydration. The primary modern treatment of severe cholera, therefore, is the replacement of fluids by intravenous infusion, Ringer lactate solution BP being fairly ideal. Lesser cases of cholera, and those improving after intravenous therapy, may be given rehydration fluids by mouth (about every 15 minutes), or via a nasogastric tube. Any of the rehydration fluids mentioned at the beginning of this section of the manual may be used, but the following formula, containing adequate quantities of potassium, is more suitable: *in 1 litre of clean water, dissolve glucose 20g, potassium chloride 1.5g, sodium bicarbonate 2.5g, and sodium chloride (common salt) 3.5g.*

In conjunction with rehydration therapy, homoeopathic remedies should be given to hasten resolution of the disease. Indeed, in many remote and impoverished places, where intravenous therapy is unavailable, the combination of homoeopathic treatment and oral rehydration may be all that there is at hand. So striking was the effect of homoeopathic therapy in the treatment of the great European epidemics of the first half of the 19th Century, that it won the greatest acclaim. In 1832, Dr F. F. Quin, a pupil of the founder of homoeopathic medicine (Dr Samuel Hahnemann), published a book entitled *Du Traitement Homoeopathique du Choléra*, in which he documented the considerable reduction of mortality associated with homoeopathic treatment, in contrast to the enormous failure of the orthodox methods of the day. We shall now consider the homoeopathic treatment in more detail:

(1) Very mild cases will be indistinguishable from *short-lasting watery diarrhoea* (see above), and should be treated similarly, with *Arsenicum album* as the key remedy.

(2) Indicated at the very onset of severe cholera, give:

> *Camphora ø (9%), 2 drops on sugar every 5–15 minutes, depending upon the favourability of reaction, for a period of 1 hour.*

{This tincture must be stored away from all other homoeopathic remedies, since it may neutralize their therapeutic effect; for similar reasons, do not get it on your hands. For persons whose weight is less than 40kg (88lb), the dose should be reduced to *1 drop*. This prescription may be hazardous to infants *less than 6 months of age*, and here should be avoided, except in dire circumstances [proceed to prescription (3), given below]. The given modern strength of the tincture, 9% [9g/100ml], corresponds to Dr Quin's recommended strength of '1:6', and should not be exceeded. The maximum number of drops allowable for an average adult in 1 hour is 24. This latter represents a total dose of camphor of approximately 54mg. With the exception of small infants, who are notoriously sensitive to even the inhalation of camphor in very small quantities, the known minimal lethal ingested dose of this substance is about 1000mg. The safety margin is, therefore, considerable.}

(3) After this period, the following remedy should be administered, the frequency of repetition being determined

by the favourability of response, and continued for some time:

Veratrum album 6 every 10–30 minutes

This remedy is strongly indicated when the patient is extremely cold, and wishes to be covered.

(4) Where muscular cramps are a dominant feature, the following remedy should be given:

Cuprum metallicum 30 every 10–30 minutes

Since the therapeutic action of *Veratrum album*, given above, will also be required, it is better to give the latter and *Cuprum metallicum* in alternation, eg:
{*Ver.alb.6*}{*15 minute gap*}{*Cup.met.30*}{*15 minute gap*}
{*Ver.alb.6*}{*15 minute gap*}{*Cup.met.30*}{*etc*}

(5) In the last stages of severe cholera, where the patient is shocked, and almost pulseless, give:

Carbo vegetabilis 30 every 10 minutes

Genus epidemicus cholerae

A remedy, or remedies, of therapeutic value with regard to *the majority* of cases during an epidemic may be used in the *prevention* of that disease in others. This is a well-defined homoeopathic tenet, and has borne much fruit in the past. Such a remedy, or remedies, constitute the so-called *genus epidemicus*. The *genus* of severe cholera is usually defined by the remedies *Veratrum album* and *Cuprum metallicum*. They may be used, therefore, in the prevention of cholera, more particularly the severe type. The value of good hygiene, however, must not be forgotten. *Veratrum album* 6 and *Cuprum metallicum* 6 should be given separately, and in alternation, at intervals of 3 days, eg:

DAY 1: *Ver.alb.6 single dose*;
DAY 4: *Cup.met.6 single dose*;
DAY 7: *Ver.alb.6 single dose*;
DAY 10: *Cup.met.6 single dose*, and so on.

This is probably the method of choice for those travelling to any area where an epidemic of cholera has broken out, or for those involved in the nursing of cholera victims. In less hazardous circumstances, the homoeopathic method suggested in *Section 3* will suffice, coupled with excellent food, water, and personal hygiene. It must be emphasised, however, that modern statistical proof of efficacy with respect to either method is presently unavailable.

Enterotoxigenic Staphylococcus aureus

Contamination of preprepared foods or milk with this bacterium may lead to the production of a harmful toxin. Some 2–6 hours after ingestion of the latter, there is a sudden onset of vomiting, followed by copious watery diarrhoea. In some cases, the diarrhoea may be almost as excessive as that found in severe cholera, and treatment should be along similar lines. Fatalities from this disorder are not unknown.

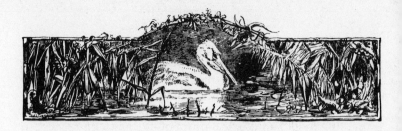

THE OVERINDULGENT TRAVELLER

Many trips are marred by overindulgence in food or alcohol, or both. In this section are discussed these matters, and the topic of potentially poisonous foods and drinks, which the traveller may be tempted to consume, but does so at his or her own peril!

Common overindulgence

The ready availability of cheap alcohol encourages many to exceed their capabilities. The immediate ill-effects of such overindulgence, which are termed *drunkenness*, include: unsteadiness, excessive jollity, lasciviousness, antipathy, aggression, hiccups, nausea, vomiting, somnolence, insensibility, and snoring. The delayed ill-effects, commonly known as *hangover*, include: headache, dry mouth, foul taste, nasal catarrh, heartburn, indigestion, constipation (more commonly), diarrhoea (less commonly), flatulence, irritability, depression, remorse, amnesia, pallor, sweating, and weakness. Severe alcoholic intoxication may even result in death. Some develop disease of the pancreas.

Alcohol may remain in the system for a considerable time after cessation of drinking, and many hours of abstinence may be required to be certain that the individual does not contravene the law with regard to driving under the influence. Pocket *calculators* are now available to assist you in computing your safety in this respect. In some countries (eg Scandinavia), regulations of this sort are even more stringent than those of the United Kingdom.

The degree to which a hangover is manifest is directly related to the quantity imbibed, the alcoholic strength of the beverage, its sugar content, and, in the case of wine, to the depth of colour, and level of postmaturity, or immaturity; the latter point also being relevant to brandies and whiskies. Non-commercial wines and spirits are particularly pernicious in their effects, because of the impurities often contained therein, which, in the case of 'home-made' spirits, may be singularly toxic. Certain types of alcoholic beverage are said to possess particular injurious properties: the headache of heavy red wines and port; the depression of gin; and the aggression of whisky. Certain drinks, when mixed, seem to be incompatible (such as cider and beer), with the production of exaggerated unpleasant symptoms; such mixing is to be discouraged. The harmful effects of alcohol are mainly attributable to its depressive action on the *brain*, its effects on the *liver*, and the production of a state of *dehydration*, by promoting the excretion of water via the kidneys. Alcohol may be damaging to the *foetus*, and should never be taken in pregnancy, except in minute quantities.

The ill-effects of alcohol may be reduced by eating before and during drinking, in order to slow its absorption into the blood. The Romans are reputed to have grown walnut trees near their permanent encampments, the fruit of which, the walnut, was believed to negate the inebriating action of wine; an attribute largely of its oil content, which, by slowing the digestive contractions of the stomach, retarded the absorption of alcohol. Such an effect can be equally achieved with virtually any other nut, be it Brazil nut, peanut, cashew, or macadamia. Nuts also provide *B vitamins*, which are highly protective of the liver (see below). Every assault upon the liver with an excess of alcohol results in a degree of damage to its cells. If such bouts of excess are infrequent (no more than once weekly), then the liver cells, which have enormous powers of restoration, are given sufficient time to return to normal function before the next onslaught. However, frequent and heavy drinking, common in expatriates, leads to progressive disturbance of the liver, which, in some cases, results in the generation of what is termed *cirrhosis*, and a premature demise therefrom. The regular consumption of foods rich in *B vitamins* is highly protective of the liver cells, and should not be forgotten. Such foods include: whole-grain products (such as brown bread, brown rice), liver, nuts, and brewer's yeast. The homoeopathic remedy *Nux vomica* is a useful corrective for minor liver cell disturbances associated with alcohol, and the remedy *Carduus marianus* should be thought of with regard to the treatment of more serious derangements of function (see below).

Since alcoholic dehydration induces many of the symptoms of hangover, it is important that it is avoided. The Continental habit of drinking bottled water along with wine at meal-times, and the North American custom of well-watering the whiskey, both do much to reduce the problem. A few glasses of clean water before retiring will also help. People with a tendency to *gout* should not allow themselves to become dehydrated, whether due to alcohol, simple lack of fluid intake, or excessive sweating, since this may precipitate an attack. This is often characterized by a sudden onset of excruciating pain in a *single* joint, usually accompanied by redness, swelling, and extreme sensitivity to touch. The consumption of excesses of red meat, veal, pork, pork products, salamis, meat extracts, kidney, liver, sweetbreads, sardines, pilchards, herrings, and anchovies, may also bring on an attack. Other common forms of *arthritis or rheumatism* may also be exacerbated by the consumption of meat, but differ from gout in that they are frequently improved by a diet *rich* in sardines, pilchards, or herrings. Gout is readily identified by means of a simple blood test, which will demonstrate a raised level of uric acid, the precipitation of which around the joints accounts for their inflammation. For some unknown reason, whole *cherries*, black or red, seem to have a preventative action with regard to gout.

They may be fresh or canned, but if the latter type are purchased, they must contain their stones. The average 'dose' is 8–10 cherries daily. The stones may be spat out, or removed just prior to eating.

Having emphasised the ill-effects of alcohol taken to excess, it should be said that, in moderation, it may have a positively beneficial action. In general, moderate intakes of alcohol stimulate appetite and digestion (especially if bitter in taste), encourage relaxation, and improve circulation (especially brandy). Moreover, certain wines would appear to be endowed with particular therapeutic properties, but should not be taken in amounts greater than 2–3 glasses daily, preferably with meals. According to the particular medical problem, so may the traveller select his wine. Table 11.1 illustrates some of these correlations.

Eating huge quantities of any food is bad, but fatty or greasy foods are particularly noxious, especially if the traveller suffers from *gallbladder disease*. Sometimes even relatively small amounts of fat or oil may induce an attack of severe pain and inflammation in the gallbladder, with accompanying nausea and flatulence. This pain is felt in the right side of the upper abdomen, and may radiate to the right shoulder or shoulder-blade. Such individuals should avoid excesses of both animal fats and vegetable oils as much as possible. These include: high-fat cheese and yoghurt, butter, fried foods, fatty meats (such as lamb, goose, and pork), cream and creamy sauces, salad dressings, oily supplements (such as cod-liver oil), pâtés, full-cream milk (skimmed is preferable), olives, nuts, and avocado pears (which are 20% oil).

Those who suffer from *recurrent indigestion*, as a result of inflammation or ulceration of the stomach or duodenum (or *hiatus hernia*), should particularly avoid: lettuce, radishes, cucumber, tomato skins, fruit skins, citrus fruits (such as oranges), Brazil nuts, tough meat, fried foods, and coffee (which, in any event, should not be taken along with homoeopathic remedies). What *should be taken*, since it is a potent healer of the stomach, is one good handful of *raw* grated cabbage (white, green, or red); this once daily *between* main meals, perhaps with a little olive oil dressing.

Table 11.1

Disorder	Recommended wine
Anaemia (iron deficiency)	Graves
Anxiety	Red Médoc
Blood pressure, high	White Sancerre, white Alsace, Pouilly
Cholesterol, high	Muscadet, Côtes de Provence
Colitis	Gaillac
Constipation	White Anjou, Vouvray
Convalescence	Red Médoc, Côtes du Roussillon
Diarrhoea (infective), in later recovery stage	Red Médoc
Gallbladder disease	White Sancerre, Pouilly
Gout[1]	White Sancerre, Pouilly, Gros Plant, Provence rosé, Saumur
Heart disease (coronary)	Dry Champagne
Indigestion[2]	Red Bordeaux, red Burgundy, Sauternes, Monbazillac
Menopause	Red Médoc, red Côte de Nuits
Rheumatism & arthritis[1]	Champagne
Urinary stones	White Sancerre, Pouilly

[1] avoid red wines and fortified wines, such as port and sherry
[2] avoid acidic or artificially carbonated white wines.

Unripe or semi-ripe fruit should be avoided, since it may induce stomach pains and diarrhoea. Unwashed and un-peeled fruit (which, in any case, is risky with regard to infective diarrhoea), when taken in large quantities, may induce diarrhoea, even if ripe, by virtue of the heavy bloom of natural yeasts.

Contrary to the usual dogmatic statements made in medical textbooks and journals, the majority of patients with *irritable bowel syndrome*, where frequent diarrhoea is a dominant symptom, fare badly on *high*-fibre diets! Such persons should avoid large quantities of bran, whole-foods (such as brown rice, and wholemeal bread), greens, fibrous fruits (such as oranges), fruit skins (which, in any case, are risky in hot climates), and beans. Fatty or oily foods should also be kept to a minimum.

Excesses of sugar are a particularly problematical for *hyperactive* children, *diabetics*, ladies prone to *thrush*, and those with *clinical hypoglycaemia* (who are always hungry).

We shall now consider the use of homoeopathic remedies in the treatment of various problems associated with overindulgence:

(1) The *key* remedy for the ill-effects of overindulgence in food in general, or alcohol (especially useful for *hangover*):

Nux vomica 30 2h

(2) For the ill-effects of *fatty or greasy* foods in particular:

Pulsatilla 30 2h

(3) For upper abdominal distention and belching:

Carbo vegetabilis 30 2h

(4) For lower abdominal distention and wind:

Lycopodium 6 2h

(5) For generalised abdominal distention and wind:

Cinchona officinalis 30 2h

(6) For intractable *hiccups*, or *abdominal cramps*:

Magnesia phosphorica 30 ½h

[cases of persistent pain in the abdomen which do not respond to simple treatments require the services of a medical professional, to exclude or confirm more serious pathology, such as acute appendicitis]

(7) For sudden attacks of *gout*, restrict to a vegetarian diet, give 24 whole *cherries* daily (the stones may be spat out), plenty of extra fluids, rest the offending joint, and administer:

(a) *Internally*:

Urtica urens ø 5 drops 4h

(b) *Externally*, apply:

Colchicum autumnale ø 4h to the skin over the joint [the latter ø must not be taken internally, and should be clearly labelled *POISON*]

(8) To help restore liver function after prolonged over-indulgence in alcohol:

Carduus marianus ø 5 drops 6h

(9) To reduce the desire or craving for alcohol:

Quercus glandium spiritus ø 10 drops 6h

Ackee poisoning (Vomiting sickness of Jamaica)

The small tree *Blighia sapida*, a native of the West Coast of Africa, is said to have been carried to Jamaica by Captain Bligh in 1793. In the West Indies, particularly Jamaica, its fruit, termed *ackee*, is highly esteemed. In West Africa it is known as *irsin*. The fruit is fleshy, of a red colour tinged with yellow, about 7.5cm in length by 5cm in width, and of a three-sided form. When ripe, it splits down the middle of each side, disclosing three shining, jet-black seeds, seated upon and partly immersed in a white, spongy substance. It is the latter part that is used for human consumption, but it contains a fairly deadly poison termed *hypoglycin*. The level of the latter is lowest when the fruit has ripened naturally upon the tree, its maturity being demonstrated by the spontaneous opening of the pod. The toxin is at its highest level in the unripe fruit. Even the properly ripened fruit, however, is unsafe to eat without proper preparation and cooking. The black seeds, which are also toxic, must be discarded, as must any pink membrane found in the substance of the potentially edible part of the fruit. The flesh must then be boiled, and the water discarded, since the latter will contain significant quantities of extracted toxin. Ackee, resembling scrambled egg, may be served with bacon or salted fish, and is available in cans. Personally, I would not trust it in any form. The effect of poisoning is to seriously lower the level of sugar in the blood. There is a sudden onset of abdominal pain, and vomiting, which symptoms then pass. 3–4 hours later, severe vomiting, convulsions, and unconsciousness occur, followed by death in up to 90% of cases within 1½-12 hours. Where it is suspected that toxic ackee has been consumed, and this is obviously more likely in small children playing near ackee trees, the patient should be made to vomit (a finger to the back of the throat will suffice). Since the poison is precipitated by alcohol, the patient may be made to drink either wine or spirits, followed by the induction of vomiting, should the latter not occur spontaneously. Transference of the patient to expert medical care is advisable. Alcoholic washouts of the stomach should be carried out, and intravenous glucose given. The homoeopathic remedy *Blighia sapida 30 ½h* may be tried as early as possible.

Cassava poisoning

The *sweet cassava (Manihot palmata)* has been cultivated in eastern equatorial South America since early times. The roots of this variety are sweet, and may be eaten raw, apparently with impunity (although opinions to the contrary have been expressed). It is, however, less cultivated than its bitter relative, which is of greater nutritional and medical importance.

The *bitter cassava (Manihot utilissima/esculenta)*, alternatively known as *manioc*, also originates from eastern equatorial South America. It was cultivated by the Indians of Brazil, Guiana, and the warm parts of Mexico long before the arrival of the Europeans, but it is now grown in many tropical countries, up to an altitude of about 1650 metres. It is a branched, hairless shrub, about 1.3–5 metres tall, with large tuberous roots. The root is bitter, and a most virulent poison when raw, but, when grated to a pulp and the poisonous juice expressed by pressure (such as pounding), it becomes edible after washing or cooking in water. The coarse meal forms *cassava*. The expressed juice, allowed to settle, deposits a large quantity of starch, which is known as *Brazilian arrowroot, or tapioca*. The boiled juice furnishes *casareep*, a condimental sauce used in the preparation of a meat stew called *pepper-pot* in Guiana and the West Indies. An intoxicating drink called *piwarrie* is brewed from the root by the Brazilians. Additional places in which bitter cassava is now found include: Africa, India, Burma, and the Philippines.

Poisoning arises from incorrect preparation of the root or its derivatives. The principal poisonous constituent is *phaseolunatin*, which yields *hydrogen cyanide (hydrocyanic acid/prussic acid/HCN)*. The effects of cyanide poisoning will depend upon the amount ingested, and physiological individuality. Sugar is said to be protective against the effects of this poison, and it has been suggested that sugar in the wine, to which had been added prussic acid, saved Rasputin from death in 1916.

Prolonged low-level ingestion of cyanide produces a variety of neurological disorders, the majority of which have been reported in either Africa or the West Indies, where bitter cassava is a staple food. The symptoms of *chronic cassava poisoning* include: paralysis, loss of sensation, blindness, and deafness. Even with treatment, the symptoms may be only partially improved. The following vitamins, of which B12 is the most important, should be used in combination (the dosages given are for adults, and should be modified for children):

(1) *Vitamin B12 (as hydroxocobalamin) 1000mcg daily (by deep subcutaneous injection) for 14 days.*

[Vitamin B12 as *cyanocobalamin* is useless]

(2) *Vitamin B1 (thiamine) 50mg 12h by mouth.*
(3) *Vitamin B6 (pyridoxine) 50mg 12h by mouth.*
(4) *Calcium pantothenate 500mg 12h by mouth.*

Acute cyanide poisoning, caused by the ingestion of larger quantities of prussic acid is a disease of sudden onset, quite different from the slowly developing condition described above. In its most severe form, unconsciousness occurs within a few seconds, and death within 5 minutes. In its lesser form, within a few minutes of ingestion, there occur dizziness, headache, staggering, enlargement of the pupils, breathlessness, and palpitations. Unconsciousness and violent convulsions follow, death often occurring within 15–60 minutes. Survival over 60 minutes is indicative of probable recovery. Emergency treatment, the medicinal side of which may not be readily available, includes:

(1) Induce vomiting, by putting a finger to the back of the throat.

(2) Maintain the air-way, and give mouth-to-mouth resuscitation if breathing stops (see *Section 18*).

(3) Give *amyl nitrite inhalations*, available in breakable glass ampoules, for 15–30 seconds each minute until intravenous therapy can be instituted. Inhalations of *ammonia* fumes, from household ammonia or smelling salts, have been suggested as an alternative, but these are highly irritant.

(4) Give intravenous *vitamin B12 (as hydroxocobalamin; not cyanocobalamin!) 50mg/kg body weight*.

> [appropriate intravenous preparations of sufficient concentration are not readily obtainable in the United Kingdom, but may be obtained from other European countries, such as France]

Obviously, the medicinal aspects of acute cassava poisoning will be restricted mainly to the domain of medical professionals.

'Pea' poisoning (Lathyrism)

Another group of nutritional plants, the *vetches (Lathyrus sativus, and allied species)*, contain cyanogens; that is to say, substances that produce prussic acid (see above). These plants produce various forms of *pea* (our own common pea is perfectly safe). These plants are used as a source of food in India, Ethiopia, and Algeria. Being more readily available during drought and famine than other foods, the symptoms of cyanide poisoning that they produce are more evident at such times of crisis. Apparently, the acute symptoms of cyanide intoxication, described above, do not occur. The disease, known as *lathyrism*, is chronic (on-going) by nature. Incontinence of urine, and impotence in males are early features, with the subsequent development of other neurological symptoms, especially paralysis. It is said to respond well to nutritional therapy, which should follow the lines given above for chronic cassava poisoning. The homoeopathic remedy *Lathyrus 6 12h* may be a useful adjunct.

Other cyanogenic foods

The seeds (kernels) of a wide variety of common fruits also yield cyanide. These include: apples (pips), cherries, plums, peaches, and apricots. Generally, an insufficient quantity is ingested to produce any illness. However, a significant number of cases of cyanide poisoning from *apricot kernels* have been reported in Turkey and Egypt.

Yam poisoning

Yams are the large, fleshy, tuberous roots of several species of *Dioscorea*, cultivated for food in tropical and subtropical countries, and weighing from 1–30kg (the average weight is 1–4kg). Yams are a principal source of a steroid precursor used in the production of the contraceptive pill. Many types, but by no means all, contain poisonous elements (especially *sapotoxins*), which, in many instances, are satisfactorily destroyed by adequate boiling. Nevertheless, there are still instances where poisoning has occurred, even after the root has been cooked! Such hazardous types include some found in Nigeria, East Africa and the Philippines, and fatalities have been recorded. Sapotoxins may cause severe diarrhoea and vomiting, and, upon absorption, may cause paralysis of vital brain centres and the heart. Symptoms can appear 30–45 minutes after a meal of yam, and coarse tremor may be a feature. The homoeopathic remedy *Dioscorea villosa 30 1/2h* may be tried in therapy, or, perhaps, an homoeopathic remedy prepared from the local strain of toxic yam, given in the same potency, and with the same frequency. Maintenance of the air-way is important in unconscious patients.

Broad bean poisoning (Favism)

Inhalation of the pollen of the broad bean plant (*Vicia faba*), or consumption of the beans themselves, may, several days after the event, result in the development of a severe anaemia, due to the destruction of red blood cells (*haemolytic anaemia*). This, however, only occurs in individuals who have a particular inherited enzymatic deficiency (*G-6-PD deficiency*). This genetic defect is commoner in those of Mediterranean origin (Greek, Semitic, Italian, etc.), and black people. The overall prevalence in whites as a whole is 1%, whereas in blacks it is about 15%. Acute haemolytic anaemia is a disease of sudden onset, with chills, fever, abdominal or back pain, pallor, jaundice, weakness, and palpitations. The urine is red or black in colour. Spontaneous recovery will often occur without special treatment, but severe cases may need transfusion of blood. Further ingestion of broad beans (or inhalation of pollen) must be avoided. Special tests are available to confirm G-6-PD deficiency. Acute haemolytic anaemia may also be precipitated in deficient individuals by many other substances, including certain orthodox antimalarial drugs, *vervain* (found in herbal sedative and Bach flower preparations), mushrooms, vitamin C supplements, and methylene blue (*Caeruleum methylenum*, used in the homoeopathic prevention and treatment of schistosomiasis).

Manchineel poisoning

Manchineel or manzanillo (Hippomane mancinella) is a tree about 9–15 metres in height found along the coastline of North, South, and Central America, as well as the West Indies, especially Barbados. Examples may also be found in East Africa. Two varieties have been described: one with holly-like leaves, the other with laurel-like leaves. Both varieties are extremely pernicious. Fruiting is profuse, and the fruits are round, and in excess of 2.5cm in diameter. They too are highly dangerous, and have been consumed by ignorant travellers and children. The sap of the tree, which resembles milk, is extremely corrosive, as are the fruits; even standing or lying beneath the tree is potentially hazardous. Contact with the skin produces a blistering eruption, and

99

contamination of the eyes leads to violent and painful inflammation (conjunctivitis). The sap should be removed from the skin or eyes with irrigations of *salt-water*. Even the smoke from the burning wood is extremely toxic. Ingestion of the fruit results in blistering and ulceration of the mouth and lips, and bloody diarrhoea with mucus (which we may term *manchineel dysentery*). Untreated, the symptoms of manchineel fruit poisoning may take up to 3 weeks to resolve, and fatalities have been recorded. In all cases of manchineel poisoning, whether affecting the skin, eyes, or digestive canal, the homoeopathic remedy *Mancinella 6 6h* may be tried, or, if this is unavailable, *Rhus toxicodendron 6 6h*.

Mexican poppy poisoning (Epidemic dropsy)

This condition has been described in India, Mauritius, Fiji, and South Africa. It is due to the sporadic contamination of *mustard oil*, commonly used in the preparation of curries, with the oil of the seeds of the *Mexican poppy (Argemone mexicana)*. The persons most frequently affected are affluent Hindu women. Its characteristics include: swelling of the legs, and, in some cases, the rest of the body; fever; diarrhoea and vomiting; pains in muscles, bones, and joints; vascular nodules of the skin, which bleed with great ease; breathlessness on exertion; weak pulse; anaemia, wasting, and extreme fatigue; and disturbances of vision, including halos around lights (epidemic glaucoma). Its symptoms resemble *beri-beri* (severe vitamin B1 deficiency), but there is no loss of sensation or paralysis. Treatment includes the following measures, given in combination (the doses stated for mother tincture and supplements are average adult doses):

(1) High protein, high calcium diet, with additional glucose.

(2) *Syzygium ∅ 3 drops 24h*, which stimulates the production of insulin by the pancreas.

(3) *Vitamin C 500mg 12h*

(4) *Rutin 50mg 12h*

(5) *Vitamin E 200IU 12h*

(6) *Argemone mexicana 6 6h*

Darnel poisoning (Lolism)

Darnel (Lolium temulentum) is an annual grass, and was formerly a common weed in European wheat-fields, from which it has now been largely eliminated. Its poisonous properties, described by Ovid and Gerard (1597), have been known since ancient times. Only the grain is toxic, containing the poison *temuline*, the presence of which is said to be due to infection with a particular fungus (although this theory has been disputed). In more recent times, darnel poisoning has been observed in Aden and Ethiopia, the contamination of wheat supplies with darnel grain being responsible. Symptoms appear about 15 minutes after ingestion, and resemble drunkenness. They include: dizziness, slurred speech, staggering, tremor, and headache. If only a small quantity has been ingested, these symptoms pass after a good sleep. Larger amounts of ingested poison produce additional symptoms: noises in the ears, impaired vision, nausea, violent abdominal cramps, diarrhoea, and the frequent passage of urine. Delirium, convulsions, coma, and death may also occur. The homoeopathic remedy *Lolium temulentum 30 ½h* may be tried.

Djenkolic acid poisoning

This occurs in Java as a result of eating a bean from the tree *Pithecolobium lobatum*. The same is said to be eaten in Burma. Unless the beans are boiled in water containing sodium bicarbonate, which effectively removes the djenkolic acid contained therein, the urinary tract becomes blocked with crystals of this substance. Symptoms include: pain in the kidney area (mid-back), painful and difficult passage of urine, and reduced or absent urinary output. Effective medical treatment includes the intravenous administration of sodium bicarbonate solution, in order to render the urine alkaline (pH8). Until such expertise is available, the following may be tried in combination:

(1) *Solidago ø 10 drops 4h* [adult dose]
(2) *Mist. pot. cit. BPC 15ml 4h well-diluted with clean water* [7.5ml 4h for children 1–5 years of age]

Castor bean and jequirity bean poisoning

Castor beans, from the plant *Ricinus communis*, found in the warmer parts of the Globe, are sometimes used to make necklaces, or other items of souvenir jewellery. They exhibit a variegated pattern of white, brown, and black. They are not normal items of food, but may occasionally be ingested, especially by children. Swallowed intact, they are harmless. If chewed, however, a poisonous substance is released, which may cause nausea, vomiting, abdominal cramps, stupor, and death. *Ricinus communis 30 ½h* may be tried. The *rosary pea, or jequirity bean (Abrus precatorius)* may also find its way into jewellery and stomachs. The bean is scarlet in colour, with a black scar indicating its point of attachment to the pod. It is not uncommon in India, Florida, Hawaii, the Caribbean, and tropical America. Its effects are similar to those of the castor bean, but, since it is less likely to be ejected by spontaneous vomiting, fatalities are more common. Try *Jequirity 30 ½h*.

Potato poisoning

The *common potato (Solanum tuberosum)* is extensively available around the World, but many are peculiarly unaware of its toxic potential. The undiseased, white or creamy tuber is wholesome enough, yet *green or sprouting* tubers, as well as the stems and leaves of the plant, contain poisonous heat-stable glycoalkaloids, which, if consumed, yield unpleasant symptoms, and, in some cases, have led to death. Ordinary cooking or boiling does nothing to protect the unsuspecting. Tubers exposed to light become green, during which process large quantities of poison are produced, and harboured in the green parts of the potato. When green, the 'eyes', skin, and young sprouts are most harmful. Symptoms of potato poisoning include: anaemia due to rupture of the red blood cells (haemolytic anaemia), red urine, loss of sensation, diarrhoea, vomiting, and stupor. *Solanum tuberosum 30 ½h* may be tried in severe cases.

Black nightshade poisoning

The *black nightshade (Solanum nigrum)* is a weed greatly distributed throughout the World. The berries, which contain numerous seeds, are usually black in colour when ripe, and are a well-known article of diet in Ethiopia. These berries contain similar poisons to those found in the green potato (see above), but the quantity contained is vary variable, depending on climate, season, and soil. They may, therefore, cause no illness, mild stomach upset, or a severe, and perhaps fatal, illness. Obviously a food to be avoided. Treatment might include *Solanum nigrum 30 ½h*.

Winter cherry poisoning

Another member of the Solanum genus of plants, the *winter cherry (Solanum pseudocapsicum)* bears small fruits resembling red cherries, which are often eaten. These, however, must be classified as mildly poisonous, in that slowing of the heart has been associated with their consumption. They should be avoided.

Pig bel (Enteritis necroticans)

Not every 'luau' is a pleasurable feast, and the type of vegetable that accompanies your meat might be a matter of life or death. The disease *pig bel* has been observed in Papua New Guinea, Indonesia, Thailand, Malaysia, and Uganda. Having a mortality rate of up to 40%, it is a severe gangrenous condition of the bowel due to a toxin produced by the bacterium *Clostridium perfringens*, commonly present in the intestines of pigs, and widely present in the soil. Normally, the toxin is destroyed by a particular digestive enzyme (*trypsin*) produced by the pancreas. However, *sweet potatoes (Ipomoea batatas)*, a common accompaniment to a feast of pork, contain a factor which inhibits the action of this pancreatic enzyme, thus allowing the bacterial toxin to exert its effect. Grand feasts of pork and sweet potato are best avoided in certain areas of the Globe. The symptoms of the disease generally appear 1–7 days after the feast, and include: vomiting, severe abdominal pain and distention, and the passage of bloody motions (in some cases). Intravenous fluids, and emergency surgery are often required. As a complement to these, consider *Pyrogen 30 4h*.

Tetrodotoxic fish poisoning

Poisoning with *tetrodotoxin* may occur after the consumption of pufferfish, porcupine fish, sunfish, globe fish, balloon fish, blowfish, and toadfish (tetrodotoxin is also found in certain newts from southern Alaska, Oregon, California, and elsewhere). The toxin is found mainly in the intestines, liver, ovaries, and skin of these fish. The novice should avoid all fish with leathery, spiny, bristly, or tuberculated skin. They are most commonly eaten in Japan, California, Australia, South America, and Africa. In Japan, specially licensed chefs prepare pufferfish as delicacies, carefully removing the toxic tissues before serving them as *fugu*. They are usually served raw, but, since tetrodotoxin is heat-stable, normal cooking would do nothing to reduce the risk. Despite the rigorous attention to detail of preparation, a number of people still suffer death by pufferfish poisoning each year in Japan. Whilst the flesh is normally safe to eat, there are times, immediately before and during the reproductive cycle, when this is not so. The effects of tetrodotoxin are primarily on the nervous system, and secondarily on the heart. The symptoms, which may occur from 10 minutes to 3 hours or more after consumption, include: numbness of the face and limbs, vomiting, salivation, sweating, headache, chest pain, and unsteadiness. Respiratory failure and death may occur in cases of severe poisoning. Professional medical assistance should be sought. Treatment includes:

(1) Induce vomiting by putting a finger to the back of the throat.

(2) Encourage excretion of the toxin by maintaining a high fluid intake.

(3) Assisted respiration will be required if respiratory failure occurs [mouth-to-mouth resuscitation may be given initially, until expert medical assistance is available].

(4) Give *Aconite 30 ¼h*.

(5) Additionally, give *Tetrodotoxin 30 ½h*.

Saxitoxic shellfish poisoning

This disease is not uncommon in the tropics. It is due to the presence of *saxitoxin* in shellfish, particularly bivalves, such as oysters, mussels, and clams, which poison they ingest from the sea-water by filtration. This toxin is particularly associated with what is termed *red tide*, a change in colour of the sea due to the presence in great numbers of particular poisonous protozoa. Unfortunately, such pernicious protozoa, whilst being present in sufficient quantities to render shellfish inedible, may not be so profuse as to produce a 'red tide'. Moreover, even though the toxic accumulation within the shellfish may take only a few days, the excretion of the poison may take several weeks. Hence, it is quite possible that even shellfish obtained in the absence of 'red tide' may be too toxic for consumption. Since saxitoxin is sensitive to heat, ordinary cooking will, however, reduce the risk of poisoning. Symptoms of poisoning after the ingestion of such shellfish may occur within a period of ½-12 hours, and are similar to those described for *tetrodotoxic fish poisoning* (see above), the mortality rate being approximately 10%. Survival for longer than 12 hours after the onset of the condition is indicative of recovery. Treatment follows similar lines to those given above for tetrodotoxic poisoning, but the homoeopathic remedy *Gonyaulax catenella 30* may be substituted, perhaps with advantage, for *Tetrodotoxin 30*. The latter remedy should, however, be used in the absence of the former.

It is to be noted that shellfish may produce 'poisoning' in two other principal ways:

(a) If inadequately cooked, and contaminated with bacteria they may give rise to *travellers' diarrhoea* (see *Section 10*).

(b) In sensitive individuals, there may be an allergic response, such as *urticaria* (nettle-rash/hives). This is discussed in *Section 16*.

Other types of shellfish poisoning have also been described, mainly affecting consumers in Japan. These include: *oyster poisoning*, due to the presence of an often deadly poison extracted from protozoa; *abalone poisoning*, due to the presence of a toxin derived from seaweed, which leads to a skin rash on exposure to light [treat with *Thuja 6 12h*]; *red whelk poisoning*, which produces paralysis [treatment includes *Curare 30 ½h*]; and *callistin poisoning*, which produces a pseudoallergic response, due to the presence of a substance resembling histamine [treat as for *mahimahi flush*, given below].

Sea urchins are sometimes served as a delicacy in the Caribbean, but must be prepared properly. The spines must be removed carefully, which may be toxic if they penetrate the skin, as must the reproductive organs, which contain another toxin which produces excessive salivation, abdominal pain, diarrhoea and vomiting [consider using the remedy *Mercurius solubilis 6 ½h*]. *Starfish* are often stated as edible, but toxicity has been reported, with the production of nausea and vomiting.

Ciguatoxic fish poisoning (Ciguatera)

Ciguatoxin is a poisonous oil, believed to originate from algae, which occasionally contaminates many species of fish in a global belt from 35°N to 35°S, and is especially found in the Caribbean and tropical Pacific. Over 400 species of fish have been found, at one time or another, to contain ciguatoxin, which renders the entirety of the flesh inedible, but those particularly implicated are the barracuda, grouper, and red snapper. Ciguatoxin is heat stable, resistant to ordinary cooking, odourless, and tasteless. The knowledge of local fishermen is indispensable with regard to the distribution of ciguatoxic fish, normally edible varieties being safe in some areas and poisonous in others. Even so, ciguatoxin may reappear in some areas of the sea, having been absent for some years, and this may only become apparent when symptoms of poisoning arise in the unsuspecting diner. Those symptoms, which arise 4–30 hours after ingestion, are, to some degree, similar to those of tetrodotoxic or saxitoxic poisoning (see above), but additional features should be noted. These include: diarrhoea, abdominal cramps, pains in muscles and joints, sleeplessness, and itching. The presence of numbness and tingling readily differentiates the condition from travellers' diarrhoea due to bacterial food-poisoning. Fortunately, death is a relatively uncommon occurrence these days, although in the past it was not so. Where death does occur, it is due to respiratory or circulatory failure. Recovery generally takes place in 1–3 weeks, but full recovery may occasionally take months or years. Sensitivity to alcohol and nicotinic acid (vitamin B3) may develop, with the production of burning sensations and reddening of the skin upon their ingestion. Allergy to seafoods may also develop. The treatment of ciguatoxic fish poisoning is similar to that described for *tetrodotoxic fish poisoning* (see above), but the remedy *Ciguatoxin 30* may be usefully substituted for *Tetrodotoxin 30*, where available.

'Mahimahi flush' (Scombroid fish poisoning)

This type of poisoning is far more common than hitherto thought, and is a direct consequence of inadequate refrigeration of certain fish after being caught. Those fish include: tuna, mahimahi, amberjack, skipjack, mackerel, bonito, albacore, and bluefish. Cooked, raw, canned, or smoked preparations of these fish have all been implicated, as has the Japanese dried fish delicacy known as *saury*. All these fish contain high concentrations of the substance *histidine* in their dark meat, which, by virtue of bacteria found on their skins, is converted to toxic *histamine*; a process which would not occur in the face of satisfactory refrigeration. The appearance, smell, and taste of the fish are usually normal, but, occasionally, there may be an unusual peppery flavour. Within minutes to several hours after ingestion, the following symptoms typically occur: *severe flushing* of the face, neck, and upper torso; headache; blistering of the mouth; difficulty in swallowing. Other possible symptoms are: itching, urticaria (nettle-rash/hives), vomiting, diarrhoea, abdominal pain, and asthma. Recovery often occurs within a few hours, but expert medical attention should be sought. Therapy includes:

(1) Induce vomiting, by placing a finger to the back of the throat.

(2) *Belladonna 30 ¼h*.

(3) In conjunction with (2), *Histaminum hydrochloricum 30¼h*.

(4) If respiratory wheezing supervenes, abandon (2), and give *Cuprum metallicum 30 ¼h* in conjunction with (3).

(5) In conjunction with any of the above measures, in order to promote toxic elimination, give *Urtica urens ø 5 drops 2h* [adult dose].

Other forms of fish poisoning

Gymnothorax poisoning may occur as the result of consuming conger, moray, or anguillid eels. Toxins are contained in the flesh, reproductive organs, and other entrails. Cooking only partially reduces toxicity. Poisoned individuals may manifest symptoms akin to *ciguatoxic poisoning*, in which case treatment will be similar (see above). Alternatively, symptoms may resemble those given for *sea urchin poisoning* (see above), treatment being similar. Respiratory support may be required.

Filefish, lampreys, and hagfish may produce toxic diarrhoea and vomiting. Herring, sprats, tarpon, and sardines may cause the same, plus toxic neurological symptoms. Mackerel, snake fish, and castor-oil fish may produce violent diarrhoea. Ratfish, elephantfish, and chimeras may depress brain activity, whilst goatfish, rudderfish, and mullet may produce hallucinations. Sawara (Japanese mackerel), ishingh (Japanese sea bass), and sandfish may cause *vitamin A poisoning*, as does polar bear liver.

Chinese and other restaurant syndromes

Up to 20% of the population are allergic to *monosodium glutamate (MSG)*. This is a popular 'flavour enhancer' used in Chinese cooking, and preprepared foods in the West. The symptoms of MSG allergy (*Chinese restaurant syndrome*), which last about 1 hour, include: flushing, burning sensation, chest pain, facial pain, headache, nausea, and vomiting. *Belladonna 30 ¼h* might be helpful to relieve. Serious complications are relatively rare. Shuddering attacks and an epilepsy-like disorder in children have been described in association with MSG ingestion. Allergic catarrh, lasting a day or so, has also been documented.

Horseradish, found in Japanese restaurants and a common accompaniment to beef in the United Kingdom, has been known to cause fainting. *Chilli*, often used in Indian, Mexican, and other schools of cookery, may produce toxic irritation to the stomach, and burning of the anus. It should be avoided by those with stomach disorders, and those suffering from piles. On the other hand, *ginger* and *cardamom* are settling to the stomach, and may be taken fairly liberally.

Bush teas

Bush teas are local infusions or decoctions of plant material, which may cause problems for the unsuspecting traveller. *Kava (yangona)* is prepared from a root throughout Polynesia as a festive beverage; overindulgence may lead to excessive excitement and weak legs ('leglessness'). *Miraa, khat, muiragi, or cafta (Catha edulis)* are alternative names for a tree in Africa, whose leaves or twigs may be infused, chewed, or smoked to produce a feeling of peace, but may induce a state of mental derangement. In the West Indies, the consumption of a brew made from *Crotalaria fulva* is implicated in the development of serious liver disease. The latter has also been caused by contamination of cereals in India with *Crotalaria* or *Heliotropium* seeds.

Some assorted hazards

Avoid all *mushrooms or other fungi* that have not been obtained from professional or experienced sources; many are poisonous, some deadly. Avoid all foods that appear mouldy; *mouldy peanuts* in Africa are implicated in cancer, whilst *mouldy maize (sweet-corn)* in Bulgaria, Roumania, and Yugoslavia has been associated with serious kidney disease. The presence of *lead* in cooking pots in Africa may lead to chronic poisoning, the level of this element being particularly high in local brews of beer. High *mercury* levels have been found in the fish of certain lakes in North America. Poisoning has occurred from the ingestion of raw or undercooked *red kidney beans*, a common ingredient of 'chilli con carne'. Serious poisoning has been recorded in Samoa from the eating of *raw sea anemones* (see *Section 15*).

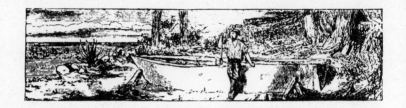

Section 12

SOME ILL-EFFECTS OF SUN AND HEAT

In this section are considered both internal and external ill-effects of sun and heat – their nature, their prevention, and their treatment.

INTERNAL DISORDERS

Heat swelling (Heat oedema/edema)

In some individuals, especially women, exposure to hot climates causes swelling of the ankles and feet, normal footwear becoming uncommonly tight. Even without treatment, this uncomfortable condition will gradually improve as acclimatisation to the new environment occurs. As discussed in *Section 5*, swelling of the ankles and feet may begin as a result of prolonged immobility during air, coach, or train travel, entry into a tropical or subtropical climate then compounding the problem. The disorder may be prevented by taking the following prescription from 24 hours prior to departure, the same being useful for treatment of the established condition:

Urtica urens ∅ 5 drops 6h

Salt and water depletion

Sweating is an important mechanism by which the body maintains its normal internal temperature, when exposed to heat. The evaporation of sweat, which takes heat from the body, is more efficient in the presence of low air humidity and wind. Humid and still environments considerably diminish the beneficial effects of sweating. Cooling is more easily achieved in the desert than in the jungle. Adaptation to hot climates may take several to many weeks, and thus may not be fully achieved by short-stay holidaymakers. Such adaptation includes: an increased ability to sweat, the conservation of salt, and an improvement in exercise tolerance. When the traveller is suddenly exposed to hot weather, sweat production progressively increases over about 6 weeks. An initial average *maximum* production of about 1.5 litres per hour becomes about 3 litres per hour at 10 days, and about 3.5 litres per hour at 6 weeks. Those who play vigorous sports in the heat, such as tennis, should note these high figures. As part of the process of acclimatisation, the concentration of salt in the sweat declines. Initial salt losses may be as much as 25g per day, but may be reduced to as little as 3g per day after 6 weeks.

The losses of water and salt must be adequately replaced. Failure to do so may result in *heat sickness* (see below). Dehydration *per se* increases the predisposition to gout (see *Section 11*), constipation (see *Section 9*), vaginal thrush (see *Section 8*), urinary infection (see *Section 8*), and kidney stones (see below). With regard to water, it is a fact that the *thirst* sensation in most people is an inadequate indicator of the state of hydration of the body, and this problem becomes more apparent when changing from temperate to hot climates. It is quite common for many people to be dehydrated and to be unaware of the problem until more serious consequences arise. Homoeopathy has documented individual variations in thirst since the 19th Century. Whilst it is true that a small percentage of persons, especially children, are excessively thirsty under all circumstances, and hence less likely to suffer heat dehydration, the majority have a

111

defective thirst mechanism, most particularly the so-called *Pulsatilla type*. Homoeopathic constitutional remedies may be administered to correct thirstlessness, with some success, especially in children, but such treatment requires the services of a professional homoeopathist. Even so, it is probably impossible to retune the thirst mechanism to a state of perfection. The majority must, therefore, rely on intellectual rather than sensorial methods for the maintenance of correct hydration. The best rule is to take sufficient fluid to maintain the urine *pale yellow* in colour, a dark brown colour signifying dehydration. As a complement to this, those indulging in intense physical exercise in hot climates can weigh themselves before and after such activity. Each kilogram of weight lost represents the loss of 1 litre of water, which should be replaced as quickly as possible, within reason. It may take 24 hours or so for this to be achieved *in toto*. Remember the old school rhyme, if you wish:

> *A pint of pure water*
> *Weighs a pound and a quarter.*

A minimum adult urinary output of 1 litre per day should be maintained.

The human *appetite for salt* is even more undependable than the sensation of thirst. Some, especially homoeopathic *Natrum muriaticum* and *Phosphorus* types, have a great desire for salt, even when the body is replete with the latter. They are unlikely to consume insufficient quantities in hot climates; unless, of course, they have been conditioned to believe that the consumption of large quantities of salt is bad for them. In many others, the appetite for salt is simply inadequate. The popular medical vogue for low-salt diets may be perfectly satisfactory in cool climates, but is positively disastrous in tropical or subtropical conditions. It has already been stated that as much as 25g daily may be required. *Salt tablets* may be used, but are inclined to cause disorders of the stomach. The addition of *half a level teaspoon of salt to every litre of liquid consumed (water, lemonade, soup, tea, etc.) or used for cooking*, is highly protective against salt depletion, without significant alteration in taste. Additional salt should also be applied to all savoury dishes.

Diuretic drugs, commonly prescribed for fluid retention and high blood pressure, favour depletion of both salt and water. It is advisable for patients undergoing such treatment to consult their own physicians before entering a hot climate.

Heat sickness (Sun sickness)

It is possible to distinguish four main types of *heat sickness (sun sickness)*:

(a) *Heat cramps*
(b) *Sun headache*
(c) *Heat exhaustion (Heat prostration)*
(d) *Heat stroke (Sunstroke)*

These will be described in detail below, together with their treatment. The factors involved in their development are as follows:

(1) **Salt and water depletion** (see above).
(2) Excessive heat (especially *humid* heat).
(3) Excessive exposure to the sun.
(4) Lack of physical fitness.
(5) Excessive exercise or physical work in sun or heat.
(6) Constitutional predisposition. Certain types of individual (eg homoeopathic *Sulphur* and *Pulsatilla* types) are more disturbed by hot environments than others (such as the homoeopathic *Silicea* type).
(7) Medical problems, such as obesity, pregnancy, heart disease, diabetes, thyroid overactivity (those with underactive thyroids fare better in heat), kidney disease. Medical advice should be sought *prior* to entry into hot countries.

Measures that will reduce the likelihood of *heat sickness* include:

(1) **Adequate salt and water intake** (see above).
(2) Artificial acclimatisation before the trip. The daily use of a *sauna* for 1–2 weeks before the trip will increase the sweating capability (and thus the cooling ability) of the body, and improve its salt conservancy. Saunas should, however, be used with proper guidance, especially where the traveller suffers from a major medical disorder.

113

(3) An exercise programme (eg weight training, cycling, swimming, keep fit) for a minimum of 2 weeks prior to departure.

(4) Severe exercise is to be avoided upon initial exposure to a hot climate. The amount of exercise taken should be gradually increased.

(5) *Alcohol* should be avoided, or strictly limited, since it significantly encourages dehydration by promoting the flow of water through the kidneys (see also *Section 11*).

(6) Adequate rest, especially after meals and exercise, and adequate sleep are desirable.

(7) Keep in the shade as much as possible, and avoid falling asleep in the sun.

(8) Appropriate clothing should be worn. It should be porous, closely woven, loose, and preferably white. Cotton is ideal, and all clothing should be changed regularly, where possible. The head and neck should be protected with porous, and preferably white headwear (eg Arab khaffieh, kepi, sombrero, straw boater). Footwear should be all-leather. Canvas or open shoes (eg sandals) are satisfactory, provided there is no risk of bites or stings from venomous creatures. Walking bare-footed is inadvisable in many places for the same reason, plus the additional risk of acquiring certain infections (eg hookworm disease). In hot and humid areas, such as jungles, wearing no clothing might seem most desirable, but this incurs the risk of insect bites, and the diseases, such as malaria, that stem therefrom.

(9) *Gustatory sweating*. Certain spices increase the ability to sweat, and thus cool the body. These include: chilli, ginger, paprika, cayenne pepper, and black pepper (see also *Section 11*). Their consumption in moderation is generally desirable in hot climates (eg in curries).

(10) *Homoeopathic constitutional treatment*, prescribed by a professional homoeopathist, may reduce the stress of heat in those prone to such problems. Ideally, this should be commenced prior to departure.

There is a fifth type of heat sickness, termed 'anhidrotic heat exhaustion', which occurs in conjunction with the skin condition known as 'prickly heat'. A full discussion of these matters will be found later in this section of the manual.

Heat cramps

These are painful spasms of the muscles of the abdomen or limbs, occurring as a result of exertion in hot climates. Involuntary muscular twitching may also occur. The following combined treatment is indicated:

(1) Give *1 level teaspoon of salt in ½ litre of water every hour for 6 hours or more*. This is the most important aspect of therapy.

(2) Gently massage the affected muscles.

(3) Give either of these two homoeopathic remedies:
   (a) *Cuprum metallicum 30 1h*
   (b) *Magnesia phosphorica 30 1h*

Sun headache

This is a throbbing headache associated with excesses of sun or heat, and is usually severe. Treat as follows:

(1) Give salt and water, as described above under *heat cramps*.

(2) Give either of these two homoeopathic remedies:
   (a) *Belladonna 30 2h*
   (b) *Glonoinum 30 2h*

Heat exhaustion (Heat prostration)

The symptoms of this condition include: confusion, weakness, dizziness, faintness, incoordination, headache, muscle cramps, overbreathing, disordered or dim vision, nausea and vomiting, and rapid, weak pulse. A bout of 'food poisoning', with diarrhoea and/or vomiting may precede and precipitate the disorder (see *Sections 10 and 11*), as indeed can any disease accompanied by nausea, vomiting, diarrhoea, or sweating (eg malaria). The skin is *cool, pale, and moist*. The oral temperature is usually normal or slightly subnormal. The differentiation between heat exhaustion and *heat stroke* is illustrated in *Table 12.1*, heat stroke being a significantly more serious medical problem.

The combined treatment of *heat exhaustion* is as follows, measures (1) and (2) being of the utmost importance!:

(1) Place the patient in a horizontal position, with legs elevated, in a shaded place.

Table 12.1

Heat exhaustion	Heat stroke
Pale, cool, sweaty skin	Red, hot, dry skin
No fever	High fever
Weakness	Very ill or unconscious
Serious condition	**Grave medical emergency**

(2) Give *salt and water*, as described above under *heat cramps*.

(3) Gently massage legs from ankle to knee.

(4) Give either of the following homoeopathic remedies:
  (a) *Carbo vegetabilis 30 ¼h [crushed/liquid form]*
  (b) *Bach Rescue Remedy ¼h*

(5) If cramps are severe, add either of the homoeopathic remedies given above, under *heat cramps*, in the same dosage.

(6) Expert medical assistance should be sought if the patient fails to respond rapidly to the above measures (see below *).

Some diagnostic problems*
In the tropics, there may be confusion between the symptoms of heat exhaustion, and those of algid malaria (see Section 20), some types of 'food poisoning', and chemical poisoning (see Sections 10 and 11), all of which may present a very similar clinical picture. Should the patient fail to respond rapidly to the measures given above, expert medical help should be sought, so that treatment along different lines may be instituted in accordance with the correct diagnosis.

Heat stroke (Sunstroke)
This is a rare but serious disorder, and requires *urgent* medical attention. It is due to failure of the heat-regulating mechanism of the body. The features of established heat stroke are outlined in *Table 12.1*. **Warning signs** of its onset include:

(1) **Diminution or cessation of sweating**.

(2) Frequency of urination.

(3) Weakness, headache, dizziness, nausea, and muscle cramps (these features are very similar to those of *heat exhaustion*, described previously; the level of sweat production is, however, different).

(4) Rise in body temperature.

Without correct treatment, after some hours, these initial warning symptoms give way to the abrupt development of established heat stroke:

(1) Vomiting, chest pain, muscle twitching, anxiety, sometimes mental derangement.

(2) The skin becomes hot and dry, and the face red.

(3) A rapid rise in body temperature, which may reach 110°F (43.3°C).

(4) Delirium, followed by coma ensues.

(5) Urinary output falls.

(6) Convulsions and projectile vomiting are grave signs, temperatures above 108°F (42.2°C) usually inducing irreversible brain damage.

(7) The pupils, which are initially contracted, become dilated.

(8) The mortality rate is up to 50%, and death is more likely in the very young or old, those with heart or kidney disease, and chronic alcoholics.

The primary objective of therapy is the reduction of body temperature:

(1) Unconscious or semi-conscious patients should be placed in the horizontal position in a cool place, and stripped of all clothing. The airway must be maintained by placing the patient on his side, and elevating the chin.

(2) Cooling must not be too rapid, and is most safely achieved by frequently wiping the entire skin with water or alcohol (or covering the patient with a wet sheet), and fanning vigorously. Cooling may be more rapidly achieved by the use of a bath of cool (*not cold!*) water, but excessive cooling is a real danger here, and the method should be reserved for more severe cases. Rectal temperatures should be taken every 10 minutes, and the cooling operation should

cease when a reading of 103°F (39.4°C) is attained. Thereafter, the naked patient should be covered with a sheet.

(3) Assist the circulation by massaging the limbs towards the heart.

(4) In conjunction with the above measures, the following homoeopathic remedies should be given in alternation (alternately) every 10–15 minutes, until significant recovery occurs:

(a) *Belladonna 30 [crushed/liquid potency]*
(b) *Carbo vegetabilis 30 [crushed/liquid potency]*

(5) Recovery is signified by a rapid fall of body temperature, and the resumption of sweating, the latter being a particularly favourable sign.

(6) The replacement of salt and water is of secondary importance compared with the need to reduce body temperature, and unless intravenous solutions are available, must wait until the patient has recovered consciousness. Oral fluids should be given along the lines given above for *heat cramps*.

Full recovery may take up to one month, with relapses being common. Ideally, the patient should be transferred to a cooler climate. Long after an episode of heat stroke, there may be reduced tolerance to hot climates, a situation which may be modified by the prescription of homoeopathic constitutional treatment by a professional homoeopathist.

Some diagnostic problems

It may be difficult to differentiate between heat stroke, falciparum malaria (see Section 20), meningitis, and pneumonia. Since heat stroke is a serious medical emergency, treatment along the lines given above should be instituted, even in the absence of a clear diagnosis. In falciparum malaria areas, simultaneous treatment for malaria should be instituted in all cases of suspected heat stroke.

Kidney stones (Urinary calculi)

The formation of urinary stones is favoured, in those prone to such things, by dehydration. Constitutional homoeopathic treatment by a professional homoeopathist, preferably *prior* to departure to hot climates, and the maintenance of a high fluid intake, will do much to prevent such inconveniences.

The classic symptomatic picture produced by such stones is termed *renal colic*. There is a sudden onset of severe pain in one loin, which often radiates around the side of the trunk into the groin, accompanied by severe sweating. Generally, the stone will move down the urinary tract, and will be passed (often with some discomfort and difficulty), whereupon the pain spontaneously disappears. Renal colic may be differentiated from severe *urinary tract infection*, in its sudden onset without warning, the absence of fever, and the lack of burning sensation on passing water. Homoeopathic treatment may be instituted to reduce pain, and favour the passage of the stone:

(1) **Drink plenty of liquids**.

(2) For *right-sided* renal colic:

   Ocimum canum 30 ¼h

(3) For *left-sided* renal colic:

   Berberis vulgaris 30 ¼h

(4) In conjunction with either of the above, the following remedy may also be given:

   Calcarea renalis 6 4h

EXTERNAL DISORDERS

There remain to be discussed those disorders of sun and heat whose overt manifestations are mainly in the skin:

(a) *Solar urticaria*
(b) *Prickly heat (Miliaria)*
(c) *Sunburn, premature ageing, and skin cancer*

Other dermatological conditions associated with tropical or subtropical climates, which stem from fungal, bacterial, or parasitic infections, are dealt with elsewhere in this manual (see *Sections 16, 17, and 22*).

Solar urticaria (Sun nettle-rash/hives)

This is often erroneously called *prickly heat*, but true prickly heat is a rather different condition, and is described subsequently. *Solar urticaria* is an itchy and raised rash involving areas of the skin exposed to sunlight, that is to say *uncovered* parts of the body. It is a form of *photosensitivity* (abnormal reaction to sunlight), and resembles the effect of being stung by nettles. It may be prevented by taking the following prescription, preferably from 24 hours prior to exposure to a sunny climate, and this should be continued for as long as such exposure persists:

> *Urtica urens* ø 5 drops 6h

> [reduce the dose for children]

The use of hypoallergenic sunblock creams on exposed parts will also help prevent this condition (see below).

Established solar urticaria may be treated as follows:

(1) Internally:
    (a) *Urtica urens* 6 2h
    (b) *Apis mellifica* 6 2h
(2) Externally, in conjunction with either of the above, the following lotion may be applied every hour or two:

> *Viola tricolor* ø 10 drops in 50ml water

Drug, chemical, and plant induced photosensitivity

In susceptible individuals, the taking of various drugs, or contact with (or consumption of) certain chemicals or plants may produce no adverse skin reaction until there is exposure to sunlight. These include: antiseptics (bithionol, hexachlorophene, halogenated salicylanilides), chlorinated hydrocarbons, coal tar and derivatives (including benzene, creosote, and pitch), dyes (including eosin, fluorescein, and methylene blue), salts of gold and silver, plant oils (angelica root, bergamot, cedar, lemon, lime, orange, sandalwood, vanillin), optical brighteners, sunblock agents (6-methyl coumarin, glyceryl-*p*-aminobenzoic acid), plants (chrysanthemum, rue, angelica, lichens, parsnip, wild carrot), drugs (chlorpromazine, tetracyclines, nalidixic acid, psoralens, diphenhydramine, sulphonamides, phenothiazines, captopril, dapsone, furosemide, naproxen). The type of skin rash produced is variable: it may be in the form of a nettle-rash (hives), an eczema, or resemble sunburn. Such sensitivity to sunlight may persist long after the offending chemical agent is no longer in or on the body. Such drug, chemical, or plant induced photosensitivity may require more complex treatment than that given above for solar urticaria, and the services of an experienced homoeopathic practitioner should be sought.

Prickly heat (Miliaria/Lichen tropicus)

In contrast to solar urticaria, described above, the rash of *true prickly heat* is largely confined to the *covered* areas of the body. It is largely due to prolonged wetting of the skin with sweat under clothing. The excessive use of ordinary soap, bathing in salt-water, and vitamin C deficiency may be contributory factors. The essential problem in prickly heat is *blockage of the sweat pores*, whilst the sweat-glands themselves continue to secrete sweat, which, finding no vent to the surface of the skin, remains confined within its substance. Characteristically, the rash has two phases:

(a) An *acute* phase, lasting about 10 days, consisting of innumerable, intensely itchy, tiny blisters (vesicles) on a red base.

(b) This gives way to a *chronic* phase, which may last for many weeks. This has the appearance of 'gooseflesh', and there is no redness or itching, and the involved skin is completely dry. The 'gooseflesh' rash may be only apparent during or after exertion, and may disappear completely on resting.

Secondary infection is a risk, with the development of pus-filled blisters (pustules), and eczema may follow a bout of prickly heat.

The condition may be prevented by a combination of the following:

(1) Avoidance of excessive exposure to heat.
(2) Clothing should be light in weight, loose, and clean.
(3) Regular bathing in non-salty water.
(4) Avoidance of ordinary soap (glycerin-based soaps are preferable).
(5) Take internally:

vitamin C 15mg/kg of body weight daily.

(6) Take internally:

Urtica urens ø 5 drops 6h

[reduce the dose for children]

(7) Regular application of the following cream to the covered areas of the body will keep the skin supple, and help prevent blockage of pores:

Cerae Lanette	*3%*
Adipis Lanae	*5%*
Paraffini Liquidi Levis	*2%*
Calendulae ø	*5%*
Conservatoris	*qs*
Aquae Rosae Triplicis	*ad 100%*

The *treatment* of established prickly heat is as follows:

(1) Remove the sufferer to cooler conditions, where possible.

(2) To prevent infection, the affected skin should be regularly cleaned with *Rose Water (triple)*.

(3) To reduce irritation, the following may be added to the *Rose Water*:

Viola tricolor ø 10 drops per 50ml

(4) Internally, give preferably both of the following remedies:

(a) *Thuja 6 12h*

[do not use potencies higher than 6]

(b) *Urtica urens ø 5 drops 6h*

[reduce the dose for children]

(5) Where infection is apparent, with the production of pustules, discontinue prescription (4a) [*Thuja*], and give the following two remedies in alternation (alternately), with an interval of 4 hours between doses:

(a) *Rhus toxicodendron 6*
(b) *Antimonium tartaricum 6*

Anhidrotic heat exhaustion

This is a disorder of heat control due to blockage of sweat glands, usually by prickly heat (see above), and is the most common major heat disorder affecting the military in both wet and dry tropics. Acute sunburn (see below), and some chronic skin diseases (such as severe eczema) may also cause blockage of the sweat pores, and give rise to anhidrotic heat exhaustion. The characteristics of the latter are: reduced exercise tolerance in heat, with exhaustion, frontal headache, dizziness, and palpitations; excessively rapid pulse and breathing; excessive sweating of forehead and face (probably compensatory), with absent or reduced sweating on the covered parts (the rash of advanced prickly heat may only be apparent during and after exertion); the rectal temperature may be raised to 38.9°C (102°F); more urine than normal may be passed; resting, especially in a cool place improves the symptoms. Progression to heat stroke (see above) may occur. Exercise should be avoided by such patients, and treatment for the fundamental skin condition instituted. Where prickly heat is responsible (as is usually the case), the measures described previously should be utilised. Additionally, restoration of sweating in the prickly heat areas may be facilitated by inducing desquamation (peeling) of the skin by repeated applications of 10% salicylic acid in 70% ethyl alcohol (having first painted a small test area to detect any undue reaction). Following desquamation, a lanolin cream, such as that described above for the prevention of prickly heat, should be applied. Where sunburn has been responsible for anhidrotic heat exhaustion, the skin should be treated along the lines given below.

Sunburn, premature ageing, and skin cancer

The effects of ultraviolet light (UVR) upon the skin are more profound if the skin is wet or oily, and diminished in accordance with the amount of inherited pigmentation. They may be classified into early and delayed changes:

   (1) Early changes:
       (a) Tanning (deposition of pigment).
       (b) Thickening of the skin (another protective process).
       (c) **Sunburn** (painful reddening of the skin, with blistering or weeping in severe cases).
   (2) Delayed changes, which mainly involve those who have had prolonged exposure to intense UVR:

       (a) Premature ageing of the skin (dryness, wrinkling,

thinning, yellowness, blackheads, whiteheads, visible blood vessels).

(b) Skin cancers. Malignant or potentially malignant skin lesions may appear years after prolonged exposure to intense UVR. The may take the form of raised lumps that easily bleed, or isolated red and scaly patches, all of which persist and grow, albeit slowly. Fortunately, they mainly spread locally, and are usually easily dealt with by simple surgical means. The *malignant melanoma* is, however, a somewhat different kettle of fish. Essentially a mole gone mad, it is largely a change seen in the flat rather than the significantly raised variety. Any pigmented mole that suddenly grows, or bleeds, or gets darker should be viewed with suspicion, and since malignant melanomata tend to spread rapidly throughout the body, urgent surgical advice is required.

Apart from the *psychological benefits* of UVR, and its ability to help in the prevention of rickets in malnourished children, *it is essentially harmful to the skin*. The acquisition of a suntan should, therefore, be carried out in a sensible and responsible manner. To this end, the following points should be noted:

(1) Limit your first day of exposure to about 20 minutes.
(2) Increase your exposure by 10 minutes for each subsequent day.
(3) Use sunblock creams to reduce the effects of UVR. These either absorb or reflect UVR, and are readily available from pharmacies. The best are hypoallergenic, and some are more cosmetically acceptable than others. The stated Sun Protection Factor (SPF) gives you an approximate idea of their efficacy in blocking the effects of UVR. An SPF of 15 implies very high protection, whilst an SPF of 2 implies fairly minimal protection. During your stay, if wish to acquire a tan safely, move gradually from high SPF applications to low. Even so, remember that to achieve proper

protection, they should be reapplied every hour or so, and certainly after swimming or exercise. Remember that buttocks and breasts require a higher SPF than other areas of the body more commonly exposed.

(4) UVR is more intense at midday.

(5) UVR becomes more intense towards the equator.

(6) UVR is more intense at higher altitudes (skiers take note!).

(7) The effects of UVR become more intense when reflected from white sand, water, metal, or snow.

(8) Light cloud, isolated cloud obscuring the sun (with largely a blue sky), and haze do little to reduce exposure to UVR.

(9) *UVR penetrates water*, and water temperature gives no guidance as to its intensity (swimmers beware!).

(10) Leaving the skin wet after swimming increases the effect of UVR.

(11) Oily preparations tend to increase the effect of UVR (hence the use of oily preparations to promote tanning).

(12) *Vitamin E* offers some protection against the ill-effects of UVR, especially with regard to sunburn and *premature skin ageing*. It is best applied as a cream (not an ointment!) on a daily basis to all exposed areas after exposure to the sun. A simple formulation is as follows:

Unguenti Emulsificantis Aquosi	*30g*
d-Alpha Tocopheryl Acetati	*600IU*

(13) Preparatory conditioning with sunbeds or sunlamps is only of marginal benefit before travelling to sunny places.

(14) Falling asleep under the sky may cause you to exceed your quota of sun for the day (or indeed for the whole trip!).

Having discussed its avoidance, the *treatment* of sunburn is along the following lines:

(1) Apply this cream *every 4 hours*:

Hyperici ø	*10gtt*
Urticae Urentis ø	*10gtt*
d-Alpha Tocopheryl Acetati	*600IU*
Unguenti Emulsificantis Aquosi	*30g*

(2) If the above is unavailable, *cold tea* or *plain yoghurt* may be used externally, as lesser substitutes.

(3) In addition to any external application, give the following internal remedy:

> *Belladonna 30 2h*

(4) Additionally, the following nutritional supplements, which may be taken together, will be found helpful:
- (a) *Vitamin E (d-Alpha Tocopheryl Acetate) 600IU 24h*
- (b) *Vitamin C 500mg 12h*
- (c) *Zinc 15mg (elemental) 24h*

[reduce these doses for children]

Botanic treatment of solar cancer

A communication from Australia suggests the possible use of the freshly expressed juice of Symphytum officinale in the treatment of early solar skin cancers presenting as red patches. The juice is applied directly to the lesion via a plaster which is changed three times daily. Claims have also been made for the direct application, several times daily, of undiluted Oleum Melaleucae Alternifoliorum.

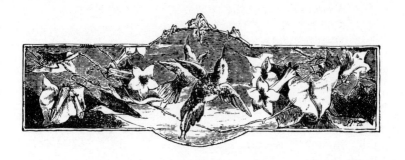

Section 13

COLD AND HIGH ALTITUDES

This section is of relevance to skiers, mountaineers, explorers, sailors, or indeed any traveller to especially cold climates.

Do not forget that even the desert may be particularly cold at night. In cold climates, remember to keep warm, dry, and moving. Beware of the effect of wind on the chilling capacity of the ambient air temperature (the *wind-chill factor*). With a blizzard blowing, an ambient *minus* 40°F (−40°C) may be converted into an effective chilling temperature equivalent to an ambient *minus* 100°F (−72°C)! At such a temperature, exposed flesh will freeze in 20 seconds, and traversing more than 100 metres on foot may prove impossible. When travelling by car in areas where such extreme conditions may arise, always carry blankets and candles. The heat from one candle alone within the passenger compartment of a car may prove life-saving. Do not leave the confines of your vehicle until either assistance arises, or the winds subside.

127

Chilling, exposure, hypothermia

Exposure of the body to cold air, or cold water may bring on muscular pains, or precipitate the overt manifestations of an incubating infection. Hence, chilling may bring on the common cold, bronchitis, pneumonia, or cystitis. Shivering is the body's way of generating extra heat, but, where this fails, the body temperature falls (*hypothermia*), and the sufferer becomes drowsy, confused, disorientated, delirious, and then comatose (unconscious). Changes in personality and comprehension in cold climates may signify hypothermia. A low rectal temperature reading (95°F/35°C or less) is confirmatory, and helps to distinguish hypothermia from *acute mountain sickness* (see after). In the case of persons rescued from cold waters, the possibility of water inhalation (drowning) should also be considered. The following measures should be instituted in all cases of suspected hypothermia before the arrival of expert medical attention:

(1) Protect from the environment (place in tent, hut, or other form of shelter).

(2) Remove all wet clothes.

(3) Cover with blankets (do *not* apply external forms of heat, such as electric blankets or hot-water bottles without expertise, since heart failure or shock may result).

(4) If conscious, give hot drinks.

(5) If unconscious, lie patient on side, with chin elevated to maintain airway, and reduce the risk of inhalation pneumonia.

(6) If conscious, give:

Aconite 30 ¼h

(7) If unconscious, give the following remedy in *¼h alternation* with *Aconite 30*:

Carbo vegetabilis 30

[remember to give remedies to unconscious patients in crushed or liquid forms]

Where exposure is a real possibility, apart from securing all possible physical protection, such as warm, wind-proof clothing, the following may be taken regularly to improve the body's resistance to cold:

> *Aconite 30 4h*

Frostbite

This is injury to the soft tissues by freezing. In mild cases the symptoms include: itching, pricking, and numbness. Superficial frostbite may be treated by removing any wet clothing, warming the affected part with a warm hand or under the armpit, and the issue of dry garments. Burning and tenderness are experienced during thawing. More severe cases may benefit from rapid thawing in stirred *lukewarm* water (not hotter than 42°C/107.6°F) for up to 30 minutes, provided that the frostbitten part can be protected from subsequent mechanical injury or refreezing. If refreezing is a distinct possibility, it is better to avoid rapid thawing techniques until circumstances change, since refreezing significantly increases tissue damage. It is better to walk on a frostbitten foot than to incur this risk. Additionally, give:

(1) *Agaricus muscarius 6 1h*
(2) Should the skin be swollen or blistered, apply the following cream sparingly to the affected area two or three times daily:

> *Cremor Calendulae 5%*

Chilblain[s] (Pernio[-nes])

This is a red, itchy, painful area on the skin of the fingers or toes, produced by exposure to cold, but without freezing of the tissues. Paradoxically, it is usually aggravated by the application of external heat. Treat as follows:

(1) Elevate the affected part, and allow to rewarm gradually in a warm environment.
(2) Do not rub the affected part or apply external heat sources.
(3) Give either of the following internal remedies:
    (a) *Rhus toxicodendron 30 6h*
    (b) *Agaricus muscarius 30 6h*
(4) In addition to either of the above remedies, the

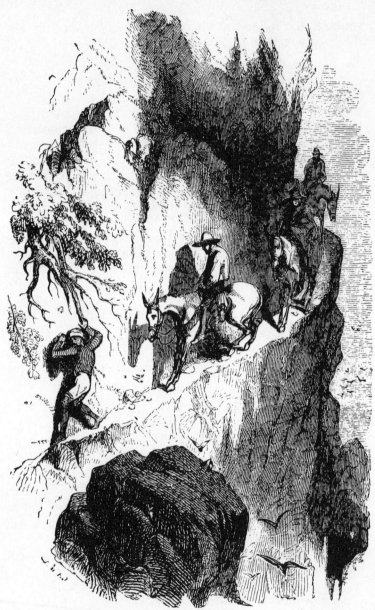

A mountain path

following *external* remedy may be gently painted on the chilblain with a fine brush or cotton-bud (it dries instantly):

    Tamus ø 12h

(5) In order *to prevent* chilblains, the following remedy is particularly useful in many cases:

    Rhus toxicodendron 30 12h

Cold urticaria

The term *cold urticaria* refers to two different entities:

(1) Familial cold urticaria, which presents as a burning sensation of the skin some 30 minutes after exposure to cold, without the appearance of a true urticarial rash (nettle-rash/hives).

(2) Acquired cold urticaria, with development of a true urticaria (nettle-rash/hives) after exposure to cold winds or water, which usually occurs in exposed areas of the skin, but may be generalised. Acquired cold urticaria may be associated with other disease (eg syphilis, glandular fever), or drug therapies (eg griseofulvin for chronic fungal infections), but, in most cases, the cause is not readily obvious. In some instances, the reaction to cold is so severe that shock, followed by death, may occur. It has, indeed, been responsible for some deaths from swimming in cold water.

For the prevention and treatment of either type, the following internal remedy should be tried:

    Urtica urens ø 5 drops 6h

    [reduce the dose for children]

Acute mountain sickness

A disorder caused by lack of sufficient time for acclimatization to the low oxygen levels of high altitudes; generally, those in excess of 2000 metres (6560 ft). Initially it is characterized by headache, weakness, drowsiness, pallor, nausea and vomiting, difficulty in breathing, and blueness of the lips and skin (cyanosis). With further evolution of the condition, there will be manifest flushing of the face, poor concentration, irritability, dizziness, noises in the ears (tinnitus), insomnia, increasing weakness, breathlessness, headaches, palpitations, and loss of weight. There is considerable variation in the tolerance of individuals to high altitudes, and those with a previous history of heart or lung disease will be at greater risk. In many instances, symptoms will disappear within 48 hours. Serious manifestations generally occur at altitudes in excess of 3000 metres (9840 ft), and often mimic those of severe pneumonia, with confusion, perhaps unconsciousness, fever, blueness of the skin, rapid pulse, wheezing (rhonchi), and rattling of fluid within the chest (râles). The following measures will be found of use in combating acute mountain sickness:

(1) Avoidance of excessive physical activity, tobacco, and alcohol.

(2) Avoidance of dehydration. Drink plenty of extra non-alcoholic fluids.

(3) Give the *mountaineer's remedy*, which promotes adaptation to high altitudes (preferably commenced before ascent):

Coca 30 6h

(4) In severe cases, the use of *oxygen* is indicated, plus removal to a lower altitude. A descent of at least 500 metres is indicated, and may be life-saving.

Where Coca fails, Cactus grandiflorus 3x-30c ½-6h may be considered in the prevention and treatment of acute mountain sickness [the lower potencies, given under medical advice, may be more effective in some cases].

Chronic mountain sickness (Monge's disease)
This is a relatively rare condition of *residents* of high-altitude communities, and is due to decompensation to low oxygen tensions. It is characterized by lethargy, blueness of the skin, depression, and clubbing of the ends of the fingers. Whilst recovery is usual on removal to sea level, those who must stay should take:

Coca 30 12h

Fear of heights
Take:

> *Argentum nitricum 30–200 4h*

Snow blindness (glare conjunctivitis)
This is painful inflammation of the eyes and light sensitivity (photophobia) due to the glare of the snow, which reflects much ultraviolet radiation. It may be avoided by the regular use of high quality dark lenses. For its treatment, see *Section 19.*

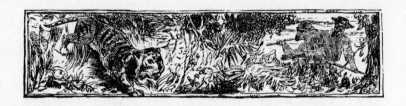

BITES AND STINGS

(INSECTS, TICKS, and MITES)

Of even greater importance than the immediate effect upon the body of insect, tick, or mite bites, is their role in the transmission of infective disease. Many of these arthropods act as *vectors*, that is to say carriers, of pathogenic organisms from animal or human reservoirs to man. Specific species of vector are usually associated with particular diseases (eg only some species of mosquito carry malaria). Even insects which do not bite, such as the common housefly and cockroach, may be instrumental in the spread of infection by the carrying of disease to food and drink. Fleas may not only transmit disease via bites, but may also cause parasitic worm infection when swallowed.

The diseases spread by arthropods may be classified as:

    (1) Bacterial [B]
    (2) Spirochaetal [S] (due to spiral bacteria)
    (3) Viral [V]
    (4) Protozoan [P] (due to unicellular parasites)
    (5) Rickettsial [R] (rickettsiae resemble bacteria, but are obliged to exist *within* the cells of the body, rather like viruses)

(6) Helminthic [H] (due to parasitic worms)

The following gives the relationship between arthropod vector and disease, together with the geographical distribution:

Diseases transmitted by mosquitoes

Yellow fever [V] Central and South America, Africa.

Dengue [V] Africa, the Americas, Pacific area, South-East Asia.

Rift Valley fever [V] South and East Africa, Egypt.

Western equine encephalomyelitis [V] USA, South Canada, Argentina.

Eastern equine encephalomyelitis [V] USA, Canada, Mexico, Cuba, Panama, Dominican Republic.

California encephalomyelitis [V] USA, especially Midwest.

Venezuelan equine encephalomyelitis [V] Northern South America, Florida, Trinidad, Panama.

St. Louis encephalitis [V] Western and Central USA, Florida.

Japanese B encephalitis [V] South-East Asia, India.

Ross River fever [V] Australia, some Pacific islands.

Malaria [P] Tropics and subtropics, with some exceptions.

Filariasis (lymphatic) [H] Tropical Africa, Asia, Australia, South America, Pacific islands.

You will note that mosquitoes do not generally transmit bacterial, spirochaetal, or rickettsial disease. Secondary bacterial infection, however, may occur at the site of a mosquito bite with the production of pus, especially in hot climates.

Diseases transmitted by ticks

Tularaemia [B] USA, Canada, Japan, Europe, Turkey.

Relapsing fever, tick-borne [S] Africa, the Americas, Mediterranean, North Africa, near East, southern former USSR.

Lyme disease [S] USA, UK, Europe, Asia, Australia.

Colorado tick fever [V] Western USA.

Russian spring-summer encephalitis [V] Former USSR.

Rocky mountain spotted fever [R] USA, Canada, Mexico, Panama, Colombia, Brazil.

Fièvre boutonneuse (including Kenya typhus, South African

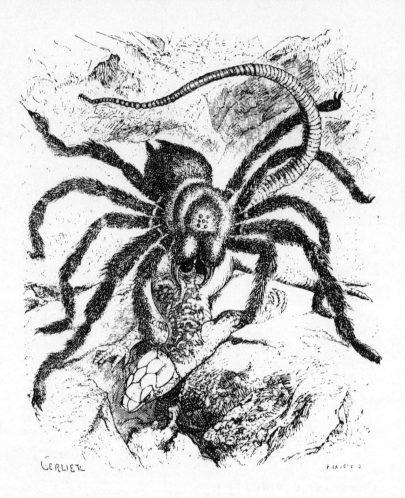

GERLIER

tick fever, and Indian tick typhus) [R] Mediterranean, Africa, India.

North Queensland tick typhus [R] Queensland (Australia).

Siberian tick typhus [R] Siberia, Mongolia.

Ehrlichiosis [R] Southeastern USA.

You will note that ticks do not transmit protozoan or hel-minthic disease, but are indeed major vectors for rickettsial diseases.

Diseases transmitted by sandflies
Bartonellosis (Oroya fever, verruga peruana) [B] Peru, Colombia, Ecuador: altitude 500–3000m.
Sandfly fever [V] Mediterranean, Middle East, Crimean coast, Azov and Black Sea, former USSR, India.
Kala-azar (visceral leishmaniasis) [P] Mediterranean, North Africa, Middle East, central Asia, China, Central and South America, India, tropical Africa.
Cutaneous leishmaniasis [P] Tropics and subtropics, Mediterranean, Middle East, North Africa, Asiatic Russia.
South American cutaneous and mucocutaneous leishmaniasis [P] Latin America.
Sandflies are a significant cause of major disease in many countries.

Diseases transmitted by other arthropods
Bubonic plague [B] (Rat fleas) Cosmopolitan.
Catarrhal conjunctivitis [B] (Eye gnats) Tropical and temperate regions, especially Egypt.
Yaws [S] (Eye gnats) Tropics.
Relapsing fever, louse-borne [S] (Human body louse) Europe, Africa, Asia.
Hepatitis B [V] (?Bed-bugs) World-wide.
African sleeping sickness [P] (Tsetse flies) West and East Africa.
Chagas' disease (South American trypanosomiasis) [P] (Kissing bugs) South and Central America, Mexico.
Epidemic typhus [R] (Human body louse) All continents except Australia.
Murine typhus [R] (Rat fleas) All continents.
Scrub typhus (tsutsugamushi disease) [R] (Larval mites). East and South Asia, western Pacific islands, Australia.
Rickettsialpox [R] (Mites) Northeastern USA.
Loiasis [H] (*Chrysops* flies) Tropical Africa, especially Congo River basin.
Onchocerciasis (river blindness) [H] (Black flies) Africa, Mexico, Central and South America.
Ozzard's filariasis [H] (Midges) Latin America.
Acanthocheilonemiasis [H] (Midges) Latin America, Africa.

Dipylidiasis [H] (Fleas, ingestion of) Europe, Asia, USA, Africa, Pacific islands.

Hymenolepiasis diminuta [H] (Fleas and cockroaches, ingestion of) India, former USSR, Japan, Italy, USA.

Remember also the role of the common housefly in the transmission of typhoid, bacillary and amoebic dysentery, cholera, and food-poisoning.

The Prevention of insect, tick, and mite bites

In this respect, the following matters must be considered:

(1) Evasion.
(2) The modification of body scent:
    (a) By internal medication.
    (b) By the use of external repellents.
(3) The use of botanic insecticides or domestic repellents, and insecticidal devices.

Evasion

Since no system of repulsion or elimination of arthropods, nor any method of immunization against their transmitted diseases is totally effective, it follows that *evasion* is the best fundamental policy for all:

(i) Wear suitable clothing. In mosquito areas wear long trousers and long-sleeved garments at night. Clothing should be of the closely-woven type, and thick enough to prevent penetration by biting insects (eg denim). The wearing of long boots, with trousers well tucked in will prevent attacks to the ankles and legs, especially with regard to mosquitoes and ticks. Dark blue clothing is attractive to *tsetse flies*, and should not be worn in the areas in which they are prevalent.
(ii) Use mosquito netting for protection during sleep.
(iii) Avoid entering heavily infested areas. Seek local advice on the matter. Ticks favour woodland, scrub, and long grass, but may also be found in 'rest-houses', market places, cattle byres, and piggeries in Africa. Mosquitoes and midges abound near water. Make enquiries concerning seasonal variations in the prevalence of various arthropods. Summer is generally the worst time for mosquitoes and wood ticks.
(iv) See also *Section 22* with regard to *sandflies*.

The internal modification of body scent
Many arthropods are attracted by the scent of their victims. Some individuals appear to be more attractive to these creatures than others. New arrivals are generally more susceptible than those who have been in residence for some time, which implies that the bodily odour changes protectively over a period of some years. The following internal remedies may be taken to induce a beneficial change in scent:

(i) Liberal amounts of *garlic* (*Allium sativum*) should be consumed, the odour of which passes to the skin. Garlic is said to be particularly repellent to ticks.

(ii) *Vitamin B1 [thiamin(e)] 50mg 12h*

   [reduce the dose for children]

(iii) *Caladium 6 12h*

Note: all three of the above measures may be used simultaneously, and continued for many months. The remedy *Ledum*, which is discussed below in relation to the prevention of excessive insect bite reaction, may be taken simultaneously with *Caladium*.

The external modification of body scent
Apart from commercially available chemicals, various plants or plant extracts may be used as insect, mite, or tick repellents. These should be applied liberally to clothing, including the socks. Additionally, application to the skin, especially around the ankles, wrists, and ears, is useful. Since allergic reactions may occur to any repellent, be it chemical or botanic, the traveller is advised to apply a small amount to a limited area of skin before general application is attempted. Persons suffering from *eczema* should be particularly cautious.

The Cherokee Indians favoured the rootstock of goldenseal (*Hydrastis canadensis*) pounded with bear grease, this bright yellow mixture being smeared over their bodies to repel insects (not a method, however, likely to appeal to the modern traveller). The Blackfoot Indians prepared a repellent from the dried flowers of the pineapple weed (*Matricaria matricarioides*). Other North American Indian botanic repellents include: an oil prepared from crushed juniper berries (*Juniperus spp.*), the blood-red juice of bloodroot (*Sanguinaria canadensis*), and the aromatic juice of American pennyroyal (*Hedeoma pulegioides*), the latter being particularly used to repel chiggers mites. The early American explorers often employed the juice from chewed tobacco leaves (*Nicotiana tabacum*).

All or any of the above might be used, and indeed may be obtained more conveniently in the form of oils or mother tinctures from homoeopathic pharmacies. However, for the purposes of the average traveller, Citronella Oil (*Oleum Citronellae/Oleum Melissae Indicum*), in view of its accepted efficacy, especially with regard to mosquitoes, is to be recommended in preference. This is a pale to deep yellow oil with a pleasant lemon-like smell, distilled from certain varieties of tropical grass (*Cymbopogon nardus* or *Cymbopogon winterianus*). Its main constituents are *citronellal* and *geraniol*. There are two main types of Citronella Oil, which differ in odour: Ceylon Oil (citronellal 10%, geraniol 30–35%), and Java Oil (citronellal 35%, geraniol 35–40%). Whilst Java Oil is more potent than Ceylon Oil, either may be used as a repellent, for which purpose it is best dissolved in 80% alcohol (1ml of oil to 4ml alcohol). This preparation may be freely applied to clothing (preferably not your best), and skin (provided there is no allergic sensitivity). In order to be effective, Citronella Oil must be applied more frequently than its chemical competitors, say every 4–6 hours (a good general rule for most botanic repellents). An alternative skin application in cream form, containing this oil, is formulated as follows (in view of its *camphor* content, it is not advisable to use it on infants less than 6 months of age):

Olei Citronellae	*18.25%*
Olei Cedri (Olei Juniperi Virginianae)	*1%*
Camphorae	*1%*
Paraffini Duri	*17.25%*
Paraffini Mollis Albi (Vaselini Albi)	*45%*
Aquae et Emulsificatoris	*ad 100%*

This cream will repel mosquitoes for 6 hours, and is also highly protective against *sandflies*. However, since it contains *camphor*, it must be kept away from homoeopathic remedies, for fear of inactivating them. Similarly, all traces of the cream must be removed from the hands before taking any homoeopathic remedies. Indeed, this course of action is advisable with regard to all aromatic substances.

An alternative antimosquito cream is based on *pyrethrum*, a relatively safe and naturally occurring insecticide, derived from the flowerheads of *Chrysanthemum cinerariaefolium* (Kenya, former Yugoslavia). With regard to mammals, absorption through the skin and toxicity are minimal, but, as with other repellents, allergic dermatitis may occur in sensitive individuals, especially those with an allergy to *ragweed* pollen. The cream is formulated as follows:

Extracti Pyrethri (40% pyrethrins)	*5ml*
Spiritus (95%)	*10ml*
Tragacanthi	*6g*
Glycerini	*6g*
Aquae	*ad 200g*

With regard to *ticks*, the above formulations may prove inadequate. Fortunately, it would seem that they are repelled by *Eucalyptus Oil (Oleum Eucalypti)*, as are fleas. It is a colourless or pale yellow oil of camphoraceous odour, obtained by distillation of the fresh leaves of various species of *Eucalyptus*. It is highly toxic when ingested, and should be carefully labelled as a *poison*. It is conveniently prepared for application to clothing and skin by dissolving it in 70% alcohol (1ml oil to 5ml alcohol). '*Lemon-scented*' *Eucalyptus Oil (Oleum Eucalypti Citriodorae)* is extracted from the leaves of *Eucalyptus citriodora* (Australia, Brazil), and contains approximately 70% of *citronellal*, mentioned above. It may be the case that this oil will prove of better service where both mosquitoes and ticks are problematical.

Against *chigger mites* (some of which transmit scrub typhus), dusting the clothing with *flowers of sulphur* is believed to offer reasonable protection.

Botanic insecticides and domestic repellents

Especially in tropical climates, there will arise the necessity to control insects and other arthropods within dwellings, tents, or camp-sites. We may use insecticidal devices (see below), repellents, or insecticides. I use the term *insecticide* loosely to encompass chemical or botanic agents destructive of both insects and other arthropods, such as ticks or mites. *Pyrethrum*, referred to previously, is truly insecticidal, but also is useful in the control of domestic ticks. Most botanic insecticides are *contact* poisons; that is to say, they act by penetration of the integument of the arthropod. They also have a short life in the environment, and generally do not cause long-term damage to the ecology. Some are very safe to man and other mammals, such as pyrethrum and *derris*, but the latter is highly toxic to fish, and should not be allowed to contaminate their waters. Pyrethrum may be purchased (from a reliable source) in the form of mosquito coils, which are allowed to burn slowly throughout the day or night within a tent or room (the vapour is not toxic to mammals). Derris powder is well-known to organic gardeners as a non-selective, short-acting insecticide, and is prepared from the dried roots of *Derris elliptica, Derris malaccensis*, or other species of *Derris* (Old World tropics). Its essential active constituent is *rotenone*. As with many other insecticides, it may cause allergic dermatitis, and inhalation is inadvisable.

Throughout the World there are in use a wide variety of botanic repellents and insecticides, of which the traveller may take advantage, out of either ecological altruism or just plain necessity. For the traveller's convenience, some of these are listed below according to their geographical location:

THE AMERICAS

Annona cherimola. Tropical. Seed resin used against lice.
Annona squamosa. Location and use as above.
Croton texensis. New Mexico. Indian insecticide.
Erigeron canadensis. North and South America (also Europe). Flea repellent. Also burnt to kill fleas, gnats.
Eupatorium capillifolium. Eastern North America. Repellent.
Eupatorium compositifolium. Location and use as above.
Funastrum clausum. Tropical. Latex strongly insecticidal.

Ipomoea quamoclit. Tropical. Seeds insecticidal.
Jacaranda filicifolia. Panama. Repellent.
Jacquemontia tamnifolia. Tropical. Seeds insecticidal.
Liquidambar styraciflua. Eastern North America. Balsam used for fumigation.
Lonchocarpus nicou. South America. Roots insecticidal (rotenone).
Lonchocarpus urucu. Location and use as above.
Lonchocarpus utilis. Location and use as above.
Mammea americana. Tropical. Roots, leaves, flowers insecticidal.
Mucuna spp. Tropical. Seeds repellent.
Nicotiana rustica. North America. Leaves insecticidal (nicotine).
Nicotiana tabacum. Location and use as above.
Patrisia pyrifera. Tropical South America. Insecticidal.
Schoenocaulon officinale. Central America. Seeds insecticidal.
Simarouba versicolor. Brazil. Bark insecticidal.
Trachelospermum stans. Mexico. Cockroach poison.

AFRICA

Calotropis procera. Widespread. Insecticidal.
Clausena anisata. Tropical. Mosquito repellent.
Dolichos pseudopachyrrhizus. Tropical. Insecticidal.
Euphorbia tirucalli. Widespread. Mosquito repellent and insecticidal. Also used in India. Latex highly irritant.
Urginia altissima. Tropical and South Africa. Somalis use liquid prepared from bulb to kill cattle flies and other bot flies.

ASIA

Adina cordifolia. India. Sap insecticidal.
Anabis aphylla. Near East. Insecticidal.
Chrysanthemum coccineum. Iran to S. Russia. Insecticidal.

Chrysanthemum marschallii. Iran. Flowerheads insecticidal.
Cynanchium arnottianum. India. Insecticidal.
Gardenia lucida. Burma. Resin repellent to flies.
Liquidambar orientalis. China. Balsam used for fumigation.
Melia azedarach. Western Asia. Fruit powder insecticidal.
Stemona burkelii. Tropical. Insecticidal.
Stemona collinsae. Location and use as above.
Stemona sessilifolia. Location and use as above.
Stemona tuberosa. Location and use as above.
Tripterygium wilfordii. China. Root insecticidal.

EUROPE

Chrysanthemum parthenium. Mediterranean. Flowerheads
   insecticidal.
Cistus ladaniferus. Mediterranean. Insecticidal gum.
Delphinium consolida. Southern Europe (& near East).
   Seed extract insecticidal.
Delphinium staphysagria. Location and use as above.
Thymus vulgaris. Widely cultivated. Fly repellent.

Note: For insecticidal purposes these plants will generally
be used in the form of dusting powders, or liquid extracts
for spraying. Always avoid inhalation and contact with skin
or eyes. Always seek local expertise before attempting to
gather, prepare, or use any of these materials.

Insecticidal devices
These devices are useful, but non-selective. Only three are
worthy of mention:

(i) *Sticky fly-papers*. Easily obtained. Light and easy to carry.
Only useful indoors.
(ii) *Mosquito lamps*. Produce a pale blue light which attracts
mosquitoes and other insects. An electrified mesh surrounding the tube fries the insect instantly, with the emission of
a loud 'zap!!'. The rate of 'zapping' gives some idea of
mosquito prevalence. May be used both indoors and outdoors, but a source of electricity is required.
(iii) The indispensable *fly-swatter*.

The local effects of insect, tick, and mite bites

The reaction to a bite is not only determined by the nature of the offending arthropod, but also by the sensitivity of the subject. In some cases the initial bite may be painless (eg Alaskan and Canadian black flies, mites), but severe reaction follows, in the form of pain, swelling, blistering and weeping of fluid (black flies), or simply an irritant dermatitis develops (mites). A few will feel generally unwell, with the development of a reactive fever. Secondary bacterial infection may then follow, with the production of pus. From the traveller's point of view, severe itching is the worst symptom. It is well worth emphasising that mosquitoes and others are quite capable of biting through thin and loosely-woven clothing.

Whilst the nature of the attacker determines the character of the reaction, the sensitivity of the subject determines the magnitude. Many people are excessively reactive to bites. Their sensitivity may be reduced, however, by means of homoeopathic remedies. For constitutional desensitization, the services of the homoeopathic practitioner should be sought. However, in a great number of cases, the following prescription, taken for the duration of a trip (and preferably from 3 days before departure), will assist in the reduction of reactivity:

Ledum 30 12h

The treatment of insect bites

All irritant bites should be treated, not merely for comfort, but to reduce the possibility of secondary bacterial infection consequent upon scratching. Such treatment, unfortunately, does nothing to reduce the risk of bite-transmitted disease.

External botanic treatments are numerous. *Touloucouna oil*, extracted from the seeds of *Carapa procera* is used in tropical areas to treat mosquito bites. *Andiroba oil*, from *Carapa guineensis*, prepared as an ointment, is successfully used in tropical America and West Africa in the treatment of insect bites. In Mexico, the leaves of *Cassia emarginata* are employed. In eastern North America, the juice of dog fennel (*Eupatorium capillifolium*) is of traditional use. The

145

Indians of the western plains of the USA used purple cone-flower (*Echinacea angustifolia*) as a general treatment for bites and stings. North American Indians also used American pennyroyal (*Hedeoma pulegioides*) to treat chigger mite bites. The latter have also been treated with the balsam from *Liquidambar styraciflua* (North America), or *Liquidambar orientalis* (China).

Homoeopathically, bites may be treated both externally and internally:

(1) Apply externally the following mixture every 1–2 hours:

> *Rumicis Crispi ø*
> *Urticae Urentis ø*
> *Ledi ø*   *aa 3.3ml*

(2) Take internally (an excellent general remedy for bites):

> *Ledum 30 4h*

(3) Alternatively, remedies may be taken which are prepared from the offending insect, eg *Pulex irritans 6 6h* for flea bites, and *Cimex 6 6h* for bed-bug bites. In order to use this method successfully, a knowledge of entomology is required. Most should content themselves with prescription (2), given above.

(4) Should a watery blister develop, consider instead:

> *Cantharis 30 2h*

(5) Where secondary infection appears, as witnessed by the formation of pus (thick, yellow discharge), discontinue the former external and internal prescriptions, and take:

> *Gunpowder 6 6h*

(6) Clean secondarily infected bites regularly with *Rose Water (triple)*, and apply wet dressings of the same.

The treatment of mite dermatitis
Mites may give rise to an intensely irritating raised skin rash (dermatitis). Initially, the internal and external measures given above with regard to the treatment of insect bites

should be instituted. However, should the dermatitis be persistent, take either of the following internally:

(1) *Sulphur 6 12h*

[do not use higher potencies or repeat more often than stated]

(2) *Bovista 6 6h*

The treatment of tick bites

Ticks do not generally bite in haste. They are often felt crawling under one's clothes before delivering the *coup de grâce*. Regular inspections of the body, and investigation of any unusual sensations in tick-infested country are well worthwhile. The actual bite of the tick may go unnoticed, and they are mainly discovered, still attached to the skin, when undressing. Ticks are slow feeders, and may remain at their site of attack for some considerable time.

For practical purposes, we may say that a tick has two main parts to its anatomy: the 'beak' (which is anchored by hooks to the skin), and the body (which fills with blood). Concerning the removal of ticks, there are two important principles to be borne in mind:

(a) The body must not be separated from the beak, since the latter will remain in the skin, with septic consequences. Under no circumstances should you attempt to crudely pull a tick from the skin.

(b) Since tick secretions may be infective, either avoid handling the tick, or wash your hands carefully after doing so.

The safest initial line for removal is to induce the tick to release its hold. This may be done in a variety of ways:

(1) Apply *tincture of iodine* to the tick body.
(2) Apply true *turpentine* to the tick body.
(3) Warm (*not* burn!) the tick body with a heat source held a few millimetres away (eg smouldering match, rope, or cigar).

Hopefully, the tick will fall off. If not, gentle traction with tweezers is indicated. Inspect the tick to ensure that the beak is present, and apply *tincture of iodine* to the bite. If there is residual irritation, treat as for insect bites (see above). Should the beak remain in the skin, it should be scraped out (or removed surgically) and tincture of iodine applied to the wound.

Venomous ticks

Whereas ticks may carry infective disease, they are seldom directly venomous. *Ornithodoros coriaceus*, however, is a notable exception. This is the *'pajaroello'* of Mexico and California. In some places its bite is feared more than that of the rattlesnake. Treatment should possibly be along the lines of that suggested for snake or spider bites (see Section 15), using a remedy prepared from the tick itself.

Tick paralysis

This is a paralytic condition caused by the bites of *female wood and dog ticks* (and possibly others, such as the *lone star tick*). It is probably due to a toxin contained within the salivary glands of the tick. The disease is generally associated with tick attachment to the head, the back of the neck, or over the spinal column. It may be confused diagnostically with poliomyelitis or peripheral neuritis. Fatalities are not unknown, but dramatic improvement usually follows within a few hours after removal of the offending tick, with full recovery in a few days.

Lyme disease

This disease, named after the town of Old Lyme in Connecticut (USA), is caused by a spirochaete (spiral bacterium), *Borrelia burgdorferi*. The disease is transmitted by ticks (*Ixodes spp.*), and is now widely distributed throughout the USA. It is also found in Europe, Asia, and Australia, but the vector is unknown in the latter case. Its recognition is of increasing importance with regard to the UK, since the number of cases reported is significantly increasing. The disease is generally contracted by walking in forests, woodland, or parks, such places being the habitat of the offending tick vector. It is convenient to divide the course of the disease into three stages, although it must be appreciated that there may be considerable overlap of the latter:

(1) *Stage 1.* Within 3–30 days after the tick bite, a characteristic *skin rash*, termed *erythema chronicum migrans*, appears in 80% of cases. This is a flat or slightly raised red rash at the site of the tick bite (generally in groin, thigh, or armpit), which expands over several days, with central clearing, so as to form a ring 5–50cm in diameter. In about 50% of the patients an *influenza-like* illness develops, with fever and muscular pains.

(2) Weeks to months later the disease may enter *Stage 2*, with the development of neurological signs (15%), such as Bell's palsy (one-sided facial paralysis), or cardiac abnormalities (8%). Rashes similar to the primary rash may appear, though they are generally smaller, and are unassociated with the site of the tick bite.

(3) Months to years later *Stage 3* may arise, characterized by chronic arthritis (60%).

Since it is most important that this disease is treated in its earliest phase (before the more serious Stage 2 develops), always seek urgent medical advice if you observe an unusual ring-like rash, especially if accompanied by influenzal symptoms.

In view of the potential seriousness of this disease, any person receiving a tick bite within its known geographical bounds should consider taking the following remedy at the earliest possible opportunity, and continue taking it for approximately one month:

Borrelia burgdorferi nosode 30 12h

Should this course of action fail, with the development of the symptoms given above, urgent medical attention is required.

Note for practitioners

I suggest that the remedies Sepia (primarily) and Tellurium (secondarily) are studied with regard to their possible homoeopathicity to Stage 1 of Lyme disease. Causticum may be helpful in Stage 2.

Hymenopterous stings

The order hymenoptera includes bees, wasps, hornets, yellow jackets, and ants. It is of particular medical importance since many of its members have the capability of delivering poisonous stings. In the case of the *honey-bee* (and some wasps), the sting is detached in the act of stinging, but the poison gland attached to the sting continues to pump venom into the wound; hence the desirability of removing the sting as soon as possible. In contrast, most wasps, hornets, and bumblebees (*Bombus spp.*) can deliver repeated stings. Remember that wasps in particular are attracted by food and drink, whether indoors or outdoors.

Stings are extremely painful events, but are only dangerous under certain circumstances:

(1) If the tongue is stung, gross swelling of this organ may occur, leading to respiratory obstruction. This is an acute medical emergency, and intubation or tracheostomy may be required.

(2) Where the victim is particularly allergic to stings (a state that worsens with each subsequent sting), generalised urticaria (nettle-rash/hives), acute asthma, or even allergic shock (collapse) may occur.

(3) Multiple stinging, even in a non-allergic person, may cause death due merely to the quantity of venom injected. It has been estimated that 500 bee stings, delivered at or about the same time, are necessary to deliver a lethal dose of venom.

The European honey-bee is a fairly pacific fellow, but not all bees are the same! The African honey-bee of equatorial and warm temperate southern Africa is more aggressive. In 1956 this species was introduced into South America, where, as a result of hybridization with local bees, there evolved an excessively aggressive strain of honey-bees (known popularly as '*killer bees*'). By 1985 they had arrived in Panama, heading North! Even the slightest disturbance near the hive induces attack, with victims sometimes being pursued for over a kilometre. The risk to humans, however, has been exaggerated, and deaths from multiple stinging are rare. The risks to livestock are, in reality, much greater. *Paper-wasps*, however, which build their nests in trees, shrubs, and under the eaves of houses, have been responsible for many deaths in the Americas. In contrast, certain South American bees are stingless (as are some other hymenopterans), but nevertheless produce uncomfortable bites by twisting their mandibles within the skin. Some inject an irritant saliva into the wound.

Whilst some ants merely bite, or squirt formic acid at their victims, others possess hazardous stings. These include: fire ants, harvester ants, and numerous tropical species. The *black bulldog ant* of Australia is said to be the most dangerous. The *fire ant (Solenopsis saevissima richteri)*, a native of South America, was accidentally introduced into the USA, where it has successfully colonized the southern states. It produces clusters of small pustules (pus-filled blisters), resembling herpes, and a general reaction that may include fever, generalised urticaria (nettle-rash/hives), and asthma. A persistent dermatitis may remain at the site of attack.

The treatment of hymenopterous stings
In general, stings produce a painful lump on the skin, which may progress to the formation of a watery blister. Treatment is indicated in order to improve the comfort of the victim, to reduce the possibility of general reaction, and to minimize the risk of secondary infection.

Numerous externally applied botanic agents have been employed to this end, many of which are the product of North American Indian medicine. These include:

Anthemis cotula (mayweed). North American folk medicine. Leaves rubbed on bee stings.

Allium spp. (wild onion and wild garlic). Dakota and Winnebago Indians, also folk medicine. Crushed bulbs applied to bee and wasp stings. Reputed to be highly effective.

Atriplex spp. (saltbush). Navajo Indians: chewed stems applied to stings of bees, wasps, ants. Zuñi Indians: dried, powdered flowers and roots mixed with saliva for ant bites, or crushed fresh flowers used for stings and bites.

Echinacea angustifolia (purple coneflower). Western plain Indians. General application for stings and bites.

151

Gutierrezia sarothrae (broom snakeweed). Navajo Indians. Chewed stem applied to stings and bites.

Lonicera sempervirens (trumpet honeysuckle). North American Indians. Chewed leaves applied to bee stings.

Nicotiana tabacum (tobacco). European and North American folk medicine. Wet leaves applied to bee stings.

Opuntia spp. (prickly pear). Texas folk medicine. Poultices of plant applied to stings and bites.

Plantago major (greater plantain). European and North American folk medicine. Leaves applied to bee stings.

Solidago rigida (stiff goldenrod). Meskwaki Indians of Minnesota. Lotion prepared from flowers applied to bee stings.

Solidago sarothrae (snakeweed). Navajo Indians. Chewed plant applied to stings of bees, wasps, ants.

For the average traveller, however, the application of *vinegar* to a bee or wasp sting should prove helpful. Remember to first remove the sting itself in the case of an encounter with the honey-bee, or some wasps. The sting should be scraped out, rather than drawn out by traction from finger and thumb, or tweezers. Traction increases the quantity of venom injected into the wound.

Internal homoeopathic treatment for stings is considered valuable, and may be usefully combined with the external remedy given below, plain vinegar applications, or any external botanic agents:

(1) Apply externally the following mixture every 15 minutes:

> *Rumicis Crispi* ø
> *Urticae Urentis* ø
> *Ledi* ø
> *Allii Cepae* ø
> *Aceti Albi*   aa 2ml

(2) Take internally (an excellent general remedy for stings):

> *Ledum* 30 ¼h

(3) Alternative internal prescriptions will depend upon the nature of the sting, eg:

    (a) Wasp stings: *Vespa crabro 30 ¼h*
    (b) Bee stings: *Apis mellifica 30 ¼h*
    (c) Fire ant stings: *Solenopsis richteri 30 ¼h*
  (4) If the patient is psychologically shocked by the bite, give either of the following remedies between doses of the principal remedy (that is to say, in alternation):
    (a) *Aconite 30*
    (b) *Bach Rescue Remedy*
  (5) In cases of physical shock (collapse), place the patient horizontally on his/her side, maintain the airway, and give either of the following *every 10 minutes* until medical assistance is available:
    (a) *Carbo vegetabilis 30*
    (b) *Bach Rescue Remedy*

[use crushed or liquid preparations]

  (6) Unlike bites, stings are not generally the vehicle of transmitted infective disease. However, especially in hot climates, scratching may result in secondary bacterial infection, with the production of pus. This situation should be treated along the same lines as those suggested previously for infected bites.

Some bites or bite-like lesions of special medical importance

Please study the following:

(i) Cutaneous leishmaniasis (see Section 22).

(ii) Mucocutaneous leishmaniasis (see Section 22).

(iii) Tropical ulcer (see Section 22).

(iv) Veld sore (see Section 22).

(v) Buruli ulcer (see Section 22).

(vi) Chagoma (see Section 26).

(vii) Kala azar (see Section 26).

(viii) Trypanosomal chancre (see Section 26).

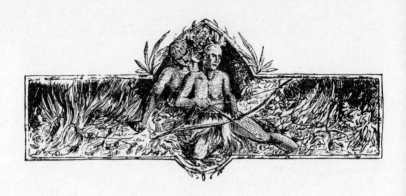

Section 15

MORE BITES AND STINGS

Having considered in Section 14 the bites and stings of insects, ticks, and mites, there remain to be discussed those of other creatures, both terrestrial and aquatic.

Snake bites
Of the 3000 or so species of snakes in the World, only approximately 10% are venomous. Tasmania is exceptional, in that all its snakes are poisonous, and, in a similarly unusual manner, in the rest of Australia venomous snakes outnumber the non-venomous. Venomous snakes are widely dispersed, but are not to be found in most Caribbean and Pacific islands (including Hawaii), Madagascar, New Zealand, Antarctica, Ireland, Iceland, Crete, and at altitudes higher than 4000m (13,000ft). The *tropics*, in particular, favour them, where they are often a *major cause of death in the native population*. Whilst some tropical islands of the Pacific and Indian Oceans may be free of venomous land snakes, their adjacent seas are the habitat of sea-snakes. The

154

latter are, however, absent from both the Atlantic and the Mediterranean.

The snake is not always successful in the injection of venom (envenoming) during the act of biting. Viewed overall, it has been estimated that over 50% of those bitten by venomous snakes escape without serious poisoning, whilst the natural mortality (in untreated cases) is somewhat less than 15%. The different species of snakes do, however, vary considerably in both the toxicity of their venom, and their ability to envenom successfully. It is pertinent to consider the main features of three principal groups.

In the case of *sea-snakes*, only about 20% of bites result in significant envenoming, but approximately 50% of those poisoned die in the absence of treatment. Whilst there are no local effects of the venom at its point of entry, severe general effects follow, with the development of muscle pains, the destruction of muscular tissue, and paralysis. The average time from bite to death is 15 hours.

With *vipers* (a group which includes rattlesnakes, moccasins, pit vipers), the situation is quite different. About 70% of bites result in significant poisoning, yet less than 20% of these cases die in the absence of treatment. Rapid swelling and pain at the point of entry are characteristic, with death of tissue (gangrene) being induced by some species. More general effects include the destruction of blood vessels, abnormal bleeding, and collapse (physical shock). The average death time is 48 hours.

With regard to *elapids* (a group which includes kraits, cobras, mambas, coral snakes), successful envenoming occurs in about 50% of bites, and of those so affected approximately 20% die in the absence of treatment, the average death time being in the order of 5–20 hours. The bites of most elapid species are not associated with any toxic signs at the point of entry, but some cobras tend to produce slow swelling, followed by tissue death (gangrene). General effects include various forms of paralysis, such as facial paralysis, and respiratory failure. The heart is also affected.

Whilst the important general properties of each group have been stated, it is important to emphasise that there may be significant differences of effect between the species of which it is comprised. Envenoming by the *Mojave rattle-snake* (southwestern USA), for example, may not be accompanied by the immediate swelling of the inflicted wound that one would normally associate with viper bites. The victim may, therefore, be lulled into a false state of optimism, only to find the development of neurotoxic symptoms (poisoning of the nervous system) some time later.

The time of the year or hour of the day may also be relevant to the assessment of risk. In North America, the peak incidence of snake bites is May to October, since snakes hibernate in the winter, and most bites occur between 2pm and 6pm. Coral snakes, however, are more active at night. In South Africa it is claimed that snake venom is more potent in the dry season than in the rainy season.

Snakes do not attack man unless they feel threatened. Sea-snakes, for example, only bite when they are handled. Always wear thick boots, socks and loose, thick trousers in snake-infested areas. Avoid walking through dense vegetation, where possible. In Africa, thumping your feet distinctly on the ground as you walk will frighten most snakes away, with the possible exception of the *puff adder*. At night, always carry a torch (flashlight) to avoid accidentally treading on a snake. Be especially cautious around log piles, crevices, caves and boulders. If sleeping in the open or in a tent, ensure that your bed is raised at least 0.3m (1ft) above the ground. If you do encounter a snake, remain still, since it will usually only attack moving objects. Unfortunately, both the *taipan* and *tiger snake* of Australia prefer to ignore this rule and may attack even a stationary person who has invaded their territory. The best thing to do is to run or, in the case of the taipan, to stand on a tree stump, a method known to the aborigines. Do not attempt to pick up a snake or even its severed head with your bare hands.

How to identify venomous snake bites

Whereas some snakes have an unusual method of delivery, such as the 'spitting cobra', the majority inject their venom via large fangs situated in the upper jaw. These are replaced at approximately monthly intervals, the reserve fangs being situated adjacently. Such fangs are absent in non-venomous species. Figure 15.1 diagrammatically illustrates typical upper jaw bite patterns.

Fig. 15.1

Bite patterns of venomous and non-venomous snakes
(upper jaw)

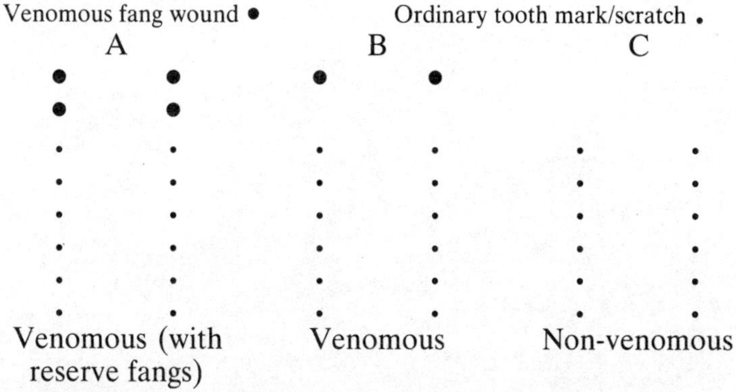

Venomous fang wound •   Ordinary tooth mark/scratch •

A   B   C

Venomous (with   Venomous   Non-venomous
reserve fangs)

Occasionally, due to inaccuracy of delivery of the attack or the intervention of clothing, only one fang wound is produced, whilst multiple strikes may produce many. Virtually all the venomous snakes which attack man are front-fanged; that is to say, the fangs are to be found in the anterior part of the upper jaw. However, some are back-fanged, with 1–3 fangs situated to the rear of each side of the upper jaw. The most important of these are the *vine (or bird) snake* and the notorious *boomslang* of South Africa, both potentially lethal to man but fortunately infrequent aggressors.

Whilst the presence of one or more fang wounds is indicative of a successful attack by a venomous snake, it does not confirm that envenoming has taken place. Since only some snakes (especially vipers) produce rapid and significant local swelling and pain, absence of these signs does not rule out poisoning. First aid treatment (see below) must be instituted immediately and the patient kept under observation for at least *10 hours*. An early transfer to specialist medical care is warranted even in an apparently symptomless case.

As will be mentioned (see below), capturing or killing the

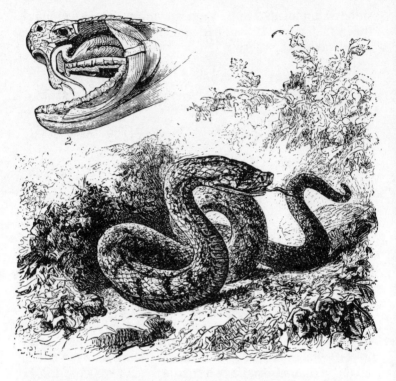

offending snake is of some considerable importance. Do not be misled by an apparent absence of fangs in the specimen, and believe that your interpretation of the appearance of the bite has been incorrect. The fangs of vipers and elapids, when not in use, are concealed by a protective membrane.

Bites from American *coral snakes* provide a difficult diagnostic problem, in that the venomous fangs are so slender that their marks are easily missed. *If you suspect a bite from such a snake, emergency treatment must be instituted even in the apparent absence of fang marks.*

It should also be realised that there may be some confusion between fang marks and skin injuries caused by thorns or cactus spines. *Always institute first aid measures when uncertain.*

First aid treatment of venomous snake bites
All bites (venomous or not) should be cleaned with a mild antiseptic, such as *Rose Water (triple)*. Most bites occur on the limbs. The *whole limb* should be tightly bandaged, and immobilized. This will limit the spread of venom. A crepe bandage is preferable, but a towel, or an item of clothing cut into a continuous strip 5–7.5cm (2–3in) wide will suffice. Incision and suction are now considered relatively ineffective, and potentially dangerous, and thus should not be used. Tourniquets should also be avoided, and reserved for the experts. Should the bite be elsewhere on the body (eg head, torso), a pad should be applied with some pressure, and, where feasible, this may be maintained by a tight bandage.

It is desirable to seek medical assistance at the earliest possible opportunity. In severe cases, the expert administration of orthodox snake *antivenin* may be considered. However, in order to select the correct antivenin, the exact identity of the attacking snake must be known. Misidentification by amateurs is not unknown, and a concerted effort must be made to capture or kill the snake, so that formal classification may be made in the medical facility. Even dead snakes must be treated cautiously.

The venom of the *spitting cobra* of Africa is delivered with great accuracy to the eyes of its victim at a maximum range of about 3m (10ft). It produces severe pain, and blindness may result. It is most important to wash out the venom immediately with the cleanest water available.

Homoeopathic treatments for venomous snake bites
In addition to the measures given above, *internal* homoeopathic treatment should be instituted in all cases of suspected or actual envenoming:

(1) Excessive anxiety in the victim tends to accelerate the spread of venom throughout the body, and verbal reassurance may be complemented by the administration of either of the following remedies as soon as possible:
(a) *Aconite 30*
(b) *Bach Rescue Remedy*

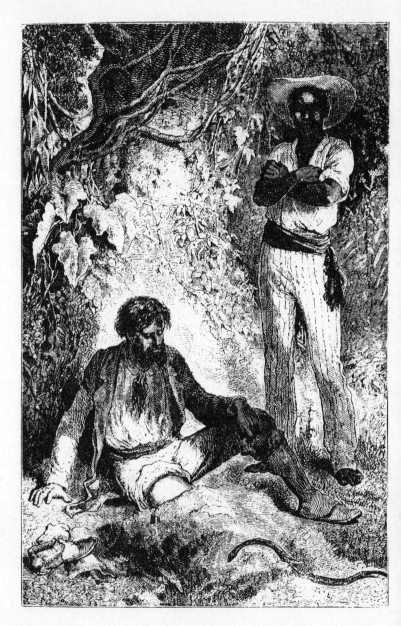

Compression & immobilization by interment

[additional doses of either remedy may be given $\frac{1}{4}h$ between doses of other indicated remedies]

(2) In an attempt to restrict the dispersion of venom, give the following immediately after the first dose of the above:

Ledum 30

(3) A few minutes after the administration of the above remedies, give the first dose of homoeopathic antitoxic treatment (by mouth). For a bite in Panama, by way of example, you would give:

Toxicaserpentium (Mexico/Central America) 30

This remedy should be given every 15 minutes, even if symptoms of poisoning are absent. In the absence of local or general symptoms, dosage should be continued for *10 hours*. If symptoms develop, it should be continued until recovery occurs. It may be combined with any indicated orthodox treatments.

Toxicaserpentium 30 is a mixture composed of individually homoeopathically prepared snake venoms appropriate to each particular area (see below for formulations). The particular variety of this remedy you will require will depend on your zone of travel, since the species of snakes encountered will differ considerably. *Toxicaserpentium (Mexico/Central America) 30* will not be appropriate for an excursion to China, where you will need *Toxicaserpentium (Far East) 30*. Whilst it is true that a case of snake bite may be treated with an homoeopathic preparation of the venom of the offending snake alone, *Toxicaserpentium* is more generally useful. It allows for both lack and error of identification of the offending species, and avoids the problem of carrying many different individual antitoxic preparations. It is important, when ordering *Toxicaserpentium*, to specify your geographical areas of concern.

(4) In cases of physical shock (collapse), institute supportive measures (such as placing the patient horizontally on his/her side and elevating chin to maintain the airway, or mouth-to-mouth resuscitation in cases of respiratory arrest), and give both *Carbo vegetabilis 30 and the indicated Toxic-*

161

aserpentium together every 10 minutes [crushed/liquid preparations].

The composition of the various types of Toxicaserpentium is given below for the benefit of the homoeopathic pharmacist. It is important that each constituent venom is potentized individually to 30c before the mixture is made. Those marked with an asterisk (*) are the more important components, in that they correspond to those venoms which commonly cause serious poisoning, whilst the remainder are less common causes, yet still potentially dangerous. You will notice that there is some overlap in their formulation. Potencies of minor venoms have been omitted [except in the case of Europe], in order to keep the number of constituents in each mixture to a level where mutual antidotal action is unlikely to occur. Whether complete or not, the composition should be stated on the label, or in any companion leaflet.

Toxicaserpentium (USA/Canada) 30
Agkistrodon piscivorus 30*   Crotalus adamanteus 30*   Crotalus atrox 30*
Crotalus scutulatus 30   Crotalus viridis 30*   Micrurus fulvius 30
Heloderma suspectum 30
  [lizard]

Toxicaserpentium (Mexico/Central America) 30
Agkistrodon bilineatus 30   Bothrops atrox 30*   Crotalux atrox 30*
Crotalus basiliscus 30*   Crotalus durissus 30*   Crotalus molossus 30
Crotalus triseriatus 30   Crotalus polystictus 30   Crotalus scutulatus 30
Lachesis muta 30   Micrurus nigrocinctus 30   Heloderma horridum 30
  [lizard]

Toxicaserpentium (South America) 30
Bothrops alternatus 30   Bothrops atrox 30*   Bothrops jararaca 30*
Bothrops jararacussu 30   Bothrops neuwiedi 30*   Crotalus durissus 30*
Crotalus durissus terrificus 30*   Lachesis muta 30   Micrurus corallinus 30
Micrurus lemniscatus 30   Micrurus mipartitus 30

Toxicaserpentium (Africa) 30
Atractaspis sp. 30   Bitis arietans 30*   Bitis gabonica 30
Dendroaspis polylepis 30   Dispholidus typus 30   Echis carinatus 30*
Naja haje 30   Naja mossambica 30*   Naja nigricollis 30*
Naja nivea 30   Thelotornis kirtlandii 30

Toxicaserpentium (Near/Middle East) 30
Atractaspis sp. 30   Bitis arietans 30*   Echis carinatus 30*
Echis coloratus 30   Naja haje 30   Naja naja 30*
Vipera lebetina 30*   Vipera xanthina 30*

Toxicaserpentium (South-East Asia) 30
Agkistrodon rhodostoma 30*   Bungarus caeruleus 30   Echis carinatus 30*
Enhydrina schistosa 30*   Hydrophis cyanocinctus 30   Lapemis hardwicki 30

| Naja naja 30* | Ophiophagus hannah 30 | Trimeresurus purpureomaculatus 30 |
| Vipera russelli 30* | | |

Toxicaserpentium (Far East) 30
Agkistrodon acutus 30	Bungarus multicinctus 30	Hydrophis cyanocinctus 30
Lapemis hardwicki 30	Naja naja 30*	Ophiophagus hannah 30
Trimeresurus flavoviridis 30*	Trimeresurus mucrosquamatus 30*	

Toxicaserpentium (Australia/Pacific Islands) 30
Acanthophis antarcticus 30*	Austrelaps superba 30	Notechis scutatus 30*
Oxyuranus scutellatus 30	Pseudechis australis 30	Pseudechis papuanus 30
Pseudonaja textilis 30*	Tropidechis carinatus 30	

Toxicaserpentium (Europe) 30
[The only snake of great concern is Vipera lebetina, but Vipera ammodytes, Vipera aspis and Vipera berus commonly cause bites, usually without serious consequences]
| Vipera ammodytes 30 | Vipera aspis 30 | Vipera berus 30 |
| Vipera lebetina 30* | | |

Botanic treatments for venomous snake bite

Numerous locally applied and internal botanic medicines have been utilised for the treatment of snake bite. Mainly out of interest, these are documented below according to their geographical area of usage:

THE AMERICAS

Antennaria plantaginifolia. Eastern North America. Rattlesnake.
Aralia spinosa. Southern USA. Root bark decoction used internally. Powdered root for wounds.
Aristolochia barbata. Brazil. Rhizome.
Aristolochia maxima. Yucatan to Venezuela. Root.
Aristolochia serpentaria. North American Indians and woodsmen. Chewed root applied to bite.
Aristolochia taliscana. Mexico. Root.
Aristolochia theriaca. Brazil. Root.
Bignonia unguis-cati. Mexico. Plant.
Blepharodon mucronatum. Central America and Mexico. Crushed leaves.
Chiococca alba. Tropical America. Plant.
Cocculus filipendula. Brazil. Possibly the fruit used.

Euphorbia polycarpa. North American Indians. Juice applied to bite, especially rattlesnake.

Echinacea angustifolia. North American plains Indians. Plant.

Fraxinus americana. Winnebago and Dakota Indians. North America. Decoction of buds drunk for rattlesnake bite. *Also used as rattlesnake repellent in boots of hunters.*

Gentiana andrewsii. Meskwaki Indians. Eastern USA. Plant.

Gymnema sylvestre. Powdered root.

Ipomoea arborescens. Mexico. Bark.

Lesquerella intermedia. Hopi Indians. North America. Chewed root applied to bite.

Machaerium angustifolium. Brazil. Gum resin.

Micania guacho. Brazil.

Penstemon spp. Navajo Indians. North America. Wet dressing of pounded leaves applied to rattlesnake bite.

Piper medium. Costa Rica. Plant.

Plumeria cellinus. Tincture used internally and externally.

Polygala senega. Seneca Indians. Eastern North America. Roots chewed and applied to bite.

Prenanthes serpentaria. Eastern North America. Root. Rattlesnake.

Ptiloria tenuifolia. Zuñi Indians. New Mexico. Powder of dried plant used internally and externally for rattlesnake bite.

Selaginella. Macerated in milk. Used internally and externally.

Simaba cedron. 'Cedron'. Seed. Used internally and externally.

Simarouba versicolor. Brazil. Bark.

Sisyrinchium. Blue-eyed grass. Tincture of plant. Used internally for rattlesnake bite.

Urechites suberecta. Tropical America. Plant.

AFRICA

Alysicarpus zeyheri. Tropical Africa. Root.
Annona nana. Angola. Root bark.

Blepharis capensis. South Africa. Plant.
Cissampelos capensis. South Africa. Leaves.
Cluytia similis. South Africa. Root.
Leonotis leonurus. South Africa. Plant.
Melianthus comosum. South Africa. Root bark or leaves.
Sebaca crassulaefolia. South Africa. Puff adder. Plant.
Trichilia capitata. Mozambique. Root.

ASIA

Arisaema speciosum. Himalayas. Root.
Aristolochia longa. Iran (to Mediterranean). Root.
Bragantia corymbosa. Java. Stems and leaves.
Cassia alata. Tropical. Leaf juice.
Clerodendron buchananii. Malaya and Indonesia. Root.
Leucas aspera. Tropical Asia. Leaves.
Leucas zeylanica. Cambodia. Boiled leaves.
Polycarpaea corymbosa. India. Leaves and flowers.
Psychotria jackii. Malaysia. Leaf.
Rhaphidophora pertusa. Indonesia to India. Black pepper.
Tabernaemontana sralensis. Indochina. Root.
Tacca fatsiifolia. Philippines and Indonesia. Plant or root.
Tacca palmata. Origin and use as above.
Uraria picta. Eastern India. Leaves.
Wrightia tomentosa. India and Pakistan. Bark.

It is extremely difficult to establish the dosage, efficacy, and safety of the above botanic medicines. No doubt they should only be used in situations of desperation, with no proper medical expertise available, and then, perhaps, only under the guidance of the knowledgeable ethnic practitioner. However, to dismiss them out of hand as nonsense would be presumptuous and unwise. There may be, after all, a few gems amongst them.

The case of *Simaba cedron (Cedron)* is worth considering in particular. In Panama the seed has the reputation of antidoting snake bites, when chewed immediately after being bitten. Dr Teste relates the story of one Hellert who was bitten by a coral snake: 'During the few seconds which it took him to take the antidote out of the little bag which he wore suspended round his neck, he was seized with violent pains at the heart and throat; but he had scarcely chewed a small portion of Cedron, of the size of a small bean, when the pain ceased as by magic. An oppression and general prostration remained. He chewed another portion of the same fruit and applied it to the wound externally, and in another quarter of an hour all he felt was a slight colic, which disappeared after eating a little. The colic was followed almost immediately by a copious evacuation of a substance that looked like curdled milk, white, with a slightly yellowish tint.'

Venomous lizard bites

Whilst there are roughly 3000 different species of lizards, only *two* are venomous! These are the *gila monster (Heloderma suspectum)* of southern Arizona and New Mexico (USA), and the *beaded lizard (Heloderma horridum)* of southwestern Mexico. These reptiles may be identified by their tuberculated skin, stumpy tails, and colouring. Gila monsters are mottled salmon pink and black, whereas beaded lizards are black and yellow. They are usually 50–75cm (20–30in) in length. Fortunately, they rarely attack man, but when they do so they bite tenaciously. Their venom is not injected into the wound, as is the case with snakes, but merely flows into it. Paralysis, difficulty in breathing, and convulsions may occur, but fatalities are extremely rare.

Treatment follows the same lines as described for *snake bite (see above)*. For gila monster bites select *Toxicaserpentium (USA/Canada) 30*, and for beaded lizard bites use *Toxicaserpentium (Mexico/Central America) 30*.

Spider bites

All spiders are venomous, their venom being injected via a pair of horny fangs. Yet, of the 30,000 or so different varieties, only a few are dangerous to man. The term *arachnidism* is applied to the poisoning effects of spider venom.

In Europe, the word *tarantula* refers specifically to *Lycosa tarentula*, a member of the family Lycosidae. Bites from

Lycosidae, with the exception of several American species, cause little discomfort, and are seldom serious. *The Russian tarantula (Trochosa singoriensis)*, whilst much feared, probably fails to deserve its reputation.

In contrast, the American term *tarantula* is casually applied to any large hairy spider found in the southern and southwest USA, or Central and South America. The bite of most of these is trivial, as is the case with the European 'tarantulas'. However, the *black tarantula of Panama (Sericopelma communis)* is decidedly dangerous, and death from its bite is not unknown. The bite of *Heteropoda venatoria*, frequently found in banana shipments, is painful but not serious.

Other South American spiders worth noting for their potential lethality are the *Brazilian huntsman (Phoneutria fera), aranha armedeira (Phoneutria nigriventer)*, the largest spider in the region, often found hiding in clothes and shoes, the *bola spider (Glyptocranium gasteracanthoides)* of Argentina, Peru, and Chile, and the *South American funnel web spider (Trechona venosa)*, although no fatalities have been recorded with respect to the latter.

An extremely important, and justifiably notorious, group of venomous spiders is that which embraces the *black widows (Latrodectus spp.)*, so named because the females, unsympathetically, tend to eat the males after mating. Various species of black widow are distributed widely throughout the warmer regions of the World. They are to be found in North and South America, southern Europe, the Middle East, the Philippines, Madagascar, South and West Africa, Australia, and New Zealand. In the USA alone there are five species: *Latrodectus mactans, L. bishopi, L. geometricus, L. hesperus, and L. variolus*. The Australian black widow *(Latrodectus hasselti)* is known as the 'red back', the New Zealand as 'night stinger', the South African as 'swart knopiespinnekop', and the Russian as 'black wolf'. Favourite haunts for these spiders are log piles, cellars, manholes, culverts, under rocks or bridges, and especially the *underside of privy seats*, a common place of attack. Indeed, the majority of bites occur in outhouses and outdoor lavatories, the male genitalia being the most popular site of attack. *It pays to lift and inspect the seat before use.*

Whereas the male black widow is a harmless creature, the female, which is larger (8–10mm long, excluding the legs), is a potent aggressor when disturbed. The bite itself is either painless, or no more than a 'pin prick'. Two tiny red spots, the fang marks, may be seen, accompanied by some local swelling. Within 10 minutes or so, severe cramping pains are experienced, which are felt in the abdomen, legs, chest, and back. By the end of an hour, the whole body is racked with unbearable constrictive pain, and the muscles become rigid, including those of the abdomen. Unfortunately, it is easy to confuse this condition with many others, such as acute appendicitis, and coronary thrombosis (heart attack), and this more so if the spider has travelled as an unwanted guest within a vehicle to an area where it would not be expected. Other symptoms, such as nausea, sweating, and difficulty in breathing, are not uncommon. Numbness and tingling of the feet may be experienced for several days. Major recovery usually occurs within 24–48 hours, but about 4% of cases die. Such an eventuality, however, is less likely if the bite is received on a limb. It has been suggested that regular creosote application within privies is helpful in preventing attacks, and those gathering logs should wear thick gloves and cover their arms.

Considerably more dangerous than the black widow is the *funnel web spider (Atrax robustus)* of Sydney, Australia, a rather large creature capable of delivering a rapidly fatal neurotoxin (nervous system poison), its attack being launched in two preferred ways. Firstly, crawling along the washing line, and pouncing upon the chest of the unsuspecting housewife hanging up her clothes. Secondly, lurking in shoes, delivering a bite to the foot. As with most types of serious envenoming, a bite to the foot is less likely to be lethal than one to the torso.

A quite different form of arachnidism is produced by the bite of the *brown recluse spider (Loxosceles reclusa)* of the southern USA, and that of *Loxosceles laeta*, found in Uruguay, Chile, and other South American countries. This is known as 'cutaneous arachnidism' or 'gangrenous spot', which latter is more descriptive. As with the black widow, the female is vastly more dangerous than the male. Most victims are bitten in the morning, and mainly in spring through to autumn (fall). The initial bite, which is said to be painless, after a period of 2–8 hours, blisters, bleeds, and then ruptures to form an ulcer, which, untreated, may enlarge for one week, and attain a diameter of 15cm (6in). The ulcer may take several months to heal, and frequently produces significant scarring and disfigurement. Other possible symptoms include fever, nausea, joint pains, and serious complications, such as fits and kidney failure.

Finally, should be mentioned the so-called *jointed spiders*, also known as 'sun spiders' or 'wind scorpions', a group found largely in tropical, subtropical, and desert regions. They are, however, not true spiders and lack poison glands. Their bite, therefore, whilst painful, is not usually serious. They are largely nocturnal in habit.

The treatment of spider bites

It is important for all those bitten by especially venomous spiders to receive urgent expert medical attention, where possible. As with *snake bite (see above)*, first aid treatment of a peripheral bite should include the application of a tight bandage to the whole of the limb, and immobilization. Orthodox treatment will include various supportive measures and, in some cases, the administration of specific *antivenin*. The muscular spasms of black widow arachnidism respond well to *intravenous calcium gluconate*. Homoeopathic treatment may be valuable, and it is appropriate to combine it with orthodox measures, according to circumstances. Homoeopathic remedies may indeed be employed for the treatment of any spider bite, whether minor or major:

(1) For minor spider bites, with minor local skin reactions only, *treat as for insect bites (see Section 14)*.

(2) For major spider bites, with severe local or general reactions (or the potential for such), *treat as for snake bites (see above)*, but substitute a remedy made from the appropriate spider for *Toxicaserpentium 30*. For example, use *Latrodectus mactans 30* for American black widow poison-

ing, *Latrodectus hasselti 30* for Australian red back poisoning, or *Atrax robustus 30* for the consequences of Australian funnel web spider attack.

In North American Indian medicine, the Navajos treated the bites of unspecified spiders with a tea of *fendler bladderpod (Lesquerella fendleri)*. The Blackfoot Indians treated the bite of a 'small brown poisonous spider' (*?Loxosceles spp.*) with a wet dressing of the pulverised flowers of the western wood lily *(Lilium philadelphicum, var. andinum)*. The latter prescription is highly intriguing, and warrants further investigation.

Scorpion stings

Of the 650 or so species of scorpion, only a few are dangerous. As most are aware, the scorpion stings from the tip of its recurved tail, which is always brought forward. The so-called 'whip scorpions' have no sting, but defend themselves with an irritant, though relatively harmless, vinegarlike fluid. Adult scorpions vary in length from about 2cm to 25cm (1–10in), the larger specimens being usually less poisonous. Many of the most venomous species are no longer than 5cm (2in). Nocturnal in habit, they rest in the day under stones, rocks, pieces of bark, logs, or even in shoes or clothing. Most scorpion stings result in no more than a sharp burning sensation at the point of entry, accompanied by pronounced swelling. Some species, however, inject largely neurotoxic venoms (nervous system poisons) which may even result in death, especially in small children. Typically, in these more serious cases, there is pain at the site of envenoming, but little swelling or redness. More important general symptoms then develop, including sweating, excessive salivation, tightness of the throat, abdominal cramps, and convulsions. Death is rare, but may occur through respiratory paralysis or other serious consequences. The five most dangerous scorpion genera are *Androctonus* (Africa), *Buthus* (Asia), *Centruroides* (southern USA and Central America), *Leiurus* (Middle East and Africa), and *Tityus* (South America). Extreme vigilance is required in Mexico (especially Durango), Brazil, Trinidad, North Africa, Egypt, Israel, India, Manchuria, and the Malayan region.

The treatment of scorpion stings

All cases of serious, or potentially serious, scorpion envenoming should receive urgent medical attention, especially in the case of small children. Where the sting has been received on a limb, the application of tight bandages and immobilization may be valuable, as with the first aid treatment of *snake bite (see above)*. Orthodox therapy may include the administration of specific scorpion *antivenins*, in addition to various supportive measures. Homoeopathic treatment may be of value, and can be combined with orthodox therapy, according to circumstances:

(1) For minor scorpion stings (local reactions only), *treat as for hymenopterous stings (see Section 14)*.

(2) For major scorpion stings, with general reactions (or the potential for such), *treat as for snake bite (see above)*, but substitute a remedy made from the appropriate species of scorpion (eg *Centruroides suffusus 30 [Mexico]*) for *Toxicaserpentium 30*).

Centipede bites

Only few centipedes have jaws sufficiently powerful to penetrate human skin. However, the American species *Scolopendra heros* and *Scolopendra morsitans*, which are 10cm (4in) or more in length, can inflict painful, yet not dangerous, bites. Some tropical centipedes, such as *Scolopendra gigantea*, some 25cm (10in) long, and *Scolopendra subspinipes*, are said to be quite poisonous, but fatalities are extremely rare. Generally the bite resembles the sting of a bee, and resolves in an hour or so, but occasionally tenderness and swelling remain for several weeks, and may be accompanied by headache, dizziness, fever, vomiting, and enlargement of the regional lymph glands. Since centipedes tend to hide in clothing and bedding at night, most people are bitten either when dressing or whilst in bed.

The treatment of centipede bites should be along similar lines to those suggested for *hymenopterous stings (see Section 14)*. Additionally, the external application of either ice or *diluted household ammonia* to the bite may produce some relief.

It is of interest to note that the Navajo Indians (USA) steeped the blossoms of *painted cup (Castilleja spp.)* and the blossoms of *penstemon (Penstemon spp.)* together in hot water, the resultant liquid being applied to the bites of centipedes; whereas the Kayenta Navajos infused that portion of the fern *Venus's hair (Adiantum capillus-veneris)* which grows above ground for the same purpose, and also for the treatment of bumblebee stings.

Leech bites

Leeches possess cutting teeth, and, once attached to their victim, secrete a substance (hirudin) which prevents the blood at the site of attack from clotting. When engorged with blood, they detach themselves, but leave behind them a wound which continues to bleed, which is slow to heal, and is especially prone to secondary infection.

Most leeches are to be found in fresh water, but some tropical species are adapted to moist terrestrial conditions. Land leeches, which are found in South America and the Far East, especially Burma, India, Assam, Malaya, Borneo, and the southwestern Pacific, are most abundant during the monsoons. They reach their human victim from the ground or via the brush, quickly finding gaps in clothing, in order to gain access to the skin. Their aquatic relatives attach themselves to swimmers, or are ingested via unfiltered drinking water. Whilst most leech attachments involve the skin, it is not unknown for aquatic forms to reach the nasal cavity, the throat, the bronchial tree, or even the bladder (expert medical attention will be needed in these unusual cases).

Leech bites are mainly painless, or responsible for minor irritation only. It follows, therefore, that their presence on the body may go undetected for some time. Multiple attachments may lead to considerable loss of blood. It is important to check carefully for leeches at frequent intervals when travelling on foot through leech-infested areas. Swimming in forest pools and streams should be avoided. *Tobacco (Nicotiana tabacum)* is said to be a good leech repellent. Either the wet leaves may be stuffed in the tops of socks or boots, or an infusion of the leaves in water may be made, the resultant dark brown liquid being applied liberally to boots, socks, and trousers.

The forceful detachment of a leech by hand may result in the mouth parts being left behind, thus increasing the risk of secondary infection. It is better to apply vinegar, salt, or a lighted match or cigar to the leech, whereupon it will detach itself completely.

Leech wounds may be treated homoeopathically, after cleaning them carefully with *Rose Water (triple)* or other mild antiseptic:

(1) To arrest bleeding, take internally:

Sanguisuga 6 ¼h

(2) To promote healing, apply the following externally 2–3 times daily (sparingly):

Cremor Calendulae 5%

(3) Should secondary infection occur, with the production of pus, apply frequent dressings (2–3 times daily) soaked in *Rose Water (triple)*, and take the following internal remedy:

Gunpowder 6 6h

Aquatic stings and envenoming

Whenever considering water sports abroad, such as swimming or sailing, always consult the locals about any risks from aquatic creatures. In Australian waters, for example, those hazards may be considerable. Fishermen and lifeguards are usually a valuable and accurate source of such information, which should seldom be ignored. Sea-snakes have been discussed previously in this section (see above).

Jellyfish stings

Jellyfish sting via their tentacles, upon which are situated numerous microscopic stinging capsules, termed *nematocysts*. Upon contact, each nematocyst discharges a small barb and a minute amount of venom into the victim's cuticle or skin. Only a few species of jellyfish are capable of inflicting serious stings upon man, the magnitude of effect depending

173

upon the size of the victim (children are more susceptible), the nature of the venom, and the quantity of nematocysts discharged.

The stings of most jellyfish result in only discomfort, tingling, and minor local swelling. The *moon jelly (Aurelia aureta)*, which occasionally causes mass panic upon beaches, including those of the UK, is typically a minor offender. The *Portuguese man-o'-war (Physalia physalis)*, found in all oceans, which possesses a main tentacle up to 30m (99ft) in length, is, however, capable of inflicting severe stings, which, upon only rare occasions, have led to death by respiratory or circulatory collapse. The local reaction is often fierce, resembling a burn, and may last a day or so. More general symptoms may include nausea, vomiting, headache, muscle pains, and shaking. Similar general symptoms to these may be produced by *Carukia barnesi* (Australia), and typically occur 10–20 minutes after being stung, the local reaction itself being quite minimal. These symptoms may persist for a day or two, but fatalities are unrecorded.

In contrast, the *box jellyfish (Chironex fleckeri)* is capable of inflicting the most deadly stings. It has, in fact, been described as 'the most venomous creature on Earth.' Breeding in the estuaries of the mangrove creeks of northern Australia, it emerges to plague the sea beaches of that region between December and July, where it is also known as the *sea wasp*. Unlike other jellyfish, it manoeuvres itself with great skill, and is never found washed up on the beach. It enters the shallows only when the sea is calm. It is highly translucent, and often goes unnoticed. It causes more deaths in Australia each year than the shark! It induces the most severe local and general symptoms, and death, due to respiratory or circulatory failure, may occur in 3–10 minutes. The pain from the sting is agonizing; its weals, like multiple poker burns, are dramatic; and residual scarring is often apparent years later.

The treatment of jellyfish stings
Jellyfish stings without lethal potential warrant only simple treatment. Should there be any adherent tentacles, they should be irrigated with liberal amounts of *vinegar*, in order

to prevent further discharge of the nematocysts, and carefully removed with a protected hand. A thick paste of *papain* powder and water should then be rubbed into the affected area of skin. Papain, an enzyme extracted from the unripe fruit of the *papaya (Carica papaya)*, is readily available as 'meat tenderizer'. Subsequently, *Cremor Calendulae 2.5% et Hyperici 2.5%* may be applied externally 3 or 4 times daily. Internal remedies, such as *Ledum* and *Aconite*, may also be given from the outset, along the same lines as suggested for the treatment of *hymenopterous stings* (see *Section 14*).

In the case, however, of *potentially lethal* stings, which are almost exclusively the domain of the *box jellyfish*, treatment must be more aggressive, and must be initiated within minutes of the attack, where possible. Remember that death, whilst not inevitable in all cases, may occur in as short a time as 3 minutes. Here, the use of *vinegar* on residual tentacles may be life-saving, in that it will limit the dose of lethal venom delivered to the patient. If vinegar is unavailable, dry sand may be applied to the tentacles before they are removed. Alcohol or methylated spirits should *never* be used, since it has been shown that these materials *increase* discharge of the nematocysts. If the major area of attack is a limb, it should be tightly bandaged in its entirety in the manner described for the treatment of *snake bites (see above)*. An orthodox specific *antivenin* is available, and should be administered by those specially trained to do so. If physical shock (collapse) occurs, mouth-to-mouth resuscitation, and external cardiac massage may be required. From the outset, homoeopathic remedies may be given, in addition to the other measures suggested, and these will be administered by mouth, preferably in a liquid form (1 drop constituting a dose). A dose of the following mixture should be given initially *every minute*, reducing the frequency as recovery ensues:

Aconite 200
Chironex fleckeri 200
Ledum 30

Should physical shock develop, change to the following mixture, giving a dose every 2 minutes:

> *Carbo vegetabilis 30*
> *Chironex fleckeri 200*

After recovery, the potential for scarring may be reduced by the twice daily external application of *Cremor Calendulae 2.5% et Hyperici 2.5% et Graphitum 8x(D8) et d-Alpha Tocopheryl Acetati (600IU per 30g)*.

The main protection against the box jellyfish is the wearing of *women's tights*, not just below, but also in a modified form to protect the upper parts of the body. These are regulation issue for the coastal life-savers of Queensland, Australia.

Other coelenterate stings

The phylum Coelenterata contains some 9000 species, of which several hundred are hazardous to man. Apart from jellyfish (see above), these include sea anemones, hydroids, and corals, widely distributed through all oceans, and possessing venomous nematocysts (see above). *Fire coral*, found in tropical oceans, has a particularly toxic venom, producing a severe sting, the discomfort of which is compounded by the multiple painful abrasions that stem from contact with its extremely sharp calcific exoskeleton. The treatment of these various stings will follow similar lines to those described above with regard to *jellyfish*.

In Samoa, the sea anemone *Matamulu (Rhodactis howesi)*, eaten raw by the indigenous population, is to be avoided when invited to dinner. Respiratory failure and death may follow its ingestion.

Venomous fish stings

The majority of fish with venomous spines are to be found in salt water; *catfish* of the genus *Pangasius*, found in the rivers of Thailand, and others found in the Amazon and elsewhere, being exceptional. Many have venomous dorsal spines, but the *stingray* is unusual in that, rather like a scorpion, it stings from the tip of the tail, which latter may also cause severe lacerations. The stingray is a placid bottom feeder, but likes to bury itself in the sand, where it may be accidentally disturbed by divers. Along the West Coast of the USA it injures about 1500 people each year. *Electric rays and eels* are not venomous, but may cause partial paralysis, or even death, by delivering significant electric shocks. The various species of *weever fish*, commonly found in eastern Atlantic and Mediterranean bays, envenom via both dorsal and gill-cover spines. Since they lie just beneath the surface of the sand, they are commonly trodden on by the unwary. Walking in the shallows with a distinct shuffle, or prodding the sand in front of you with a stick may lessen the chances of an unfortunate encounter. With spines removed, the weever will be seen offered for sale as food in Belgium and certain Mediterranean countries.

Many varieties of venomous fish are to be found in the Indian and Pacific Oceans. In addition to the stingray, should be mentioned the *lionfish, turkeyfish, scorpionfish* (common in Hawaii), *rabbitfish* (one species of which is also found in the eastern Mediterranean), and *stonefish*. The stonefish, once described by a colleague as 'the creature from the pit' (in view of its evil form), frequents coral reefs, but may also be found in estuaries and mud flats. Rather like the weever, it may go unnoticed buried beneath mud or sand. It may cause agonizing pain, and although rare, fatalities have occurred. Both the stonefish and the scorpionfish are heavily camouflaged, and may be difficult to see amongst the corals. Both are unusual for venomous fish, in that they would rather attack than retreat, even when not cornered. Whilst stingrays may inflict severe traumatic injuries, and scorpionfish local gangrene, pain rather than death is the rule for most cases of fish envenoming.

The treatment of venomous fish stings

The single most important measure for all such stings is the destruction of venom by means of wet heat, which considerably relieves the often unbearable pain. The limb should be immersed in *very hot* water (as hot as the sufferer can bear). This will generally be in the range of 110–115°F (43.3–46.5°C), and hot water must be added during the period of therapy to maintain this level of heat. After a few seconds of immersion, the pain will be greatly alleviated, and the limb must be immediately withdrawn as soon as this happens, to prevent blistering. Usually, after a few seconds, the pain returns, and the limb must once again be plunged into the hot water. Immersion in hot water with pain, and withdrawal on its significant improvement, must be alternated until pain is absent. In general this process takes about 30 minutes to complete. Where the sting has been incurred on a part other than a limb, wet heat may be applied with frequent hot towels. Additionally, and concurrently, internal homoeopathic remedies may be given along similar lines to those stated for the treatment of *hymenopterous stings* (see *Section 14*). All wounds, of course, should be inspected for spine fragments, which should be removed, and the area gently cleaned to prevent secondary infection.

Starfish and sea urchin stings

These *echinoderms* are found in all oceans. Virtually all *starfish* are harmless to man, with the exception of the *crown of thorns (Acanthaster planci)*. Whilst it is not known to attack as such, coming inadvertently into contact with it whilst diving, may leave the victim with many deep and painful puncture wounds, and other symptoms, usually short-lived, such as nausea, vomiting, and muscular paralysis.

All contact with *sea urchins* should be avoided. Even the non-venomous varieties have sharp and barbed spines that can break off after penetration of the skin, with ensuing infection. Many species of sea urchin are frankly venomous, with regard to both their spines and their jaws, and general symptoms, such as nausea, cramps, tingling, and difficulty in breathing have been reported.

With regard to echinoderm stings, whilst general symptoms are relatively unimportant, the treatment of pain and the embedded fragments is a priority. Local pain is readily treated by the application of *wet heat*, as described above for *fish stings*. Homoeopathic remedies may be used similarly. In the absence of surgical help, the problem remains concerning the treatment of the buried spines. I am assured by those familiar with such matters, that the best course of action is to hit the site of penetration with a blunt object, such as a piece of wood, in order to fragment the spines.

Following this, it would seem advisable to take internally the homoeopathic remedy *Silicea 6 6h* for a period of many weeks, or even months, in order to promote expulsion of these foreign bodies.

Molluscan envenoming

The *blue-ringed octopus (Hapalochlaena maculosa)*, which is about 10–20cm (4–8in) long, is found in shallow waters along the coast of Australia. It is not known to attack man spontaneously, but rather if it feels threatened. When angered, it exhibits iridescent blue markings. Most bites occur when visitors, ignorant of the risk, pick up this attractive creature intentionally, or inadvertently contact it whilst gathering shells. The bite delivers a potent neurotoxin, and death may occur in *a few minutes*. Treatment should be similar to that described for *box jellyfish stings* (see above), including the use of the constrictive bandage. Homoeopathic remedies may also be used in a similar manner, but substituting the remedy *Hapalochlaena maculosa 200* for *Chironex fleckeri 200* in the stated mixed formulations.

Cone shells (Conidae) are highly attractive molluscs which inhabit both sand and coral reefs in tropical and subtropical waters. The cone shell delivers its venom via an ejectable tooth contained in the end of a long flexible proboscis. Shell collectors are common victims. General symptoms include numbness, tingling, and blurred vision. In many instances, spontaneous recovery occurs in 6–8 hours, but death from circulatory collapse in 15 minutes is also not unknown. In treatment, *wet heat*, should be applied as described with regard to *fish envenoming* (see above). Additionally, homoeopathic remedies may be given in a similar way to that described for *box jellyfish stings* (see above), but substituting a remedy made from the offending species of cone shell (eg *Conus geographus 200*) for *Chironex fleckeri 200* in the stated mixed formulations, and using the first of the latter with less frequent repetition (initially, one dose every 5 minutes).

It should be emphasised that in all cases of potentially serious aquatic envenoming, local expert assistance should be sought

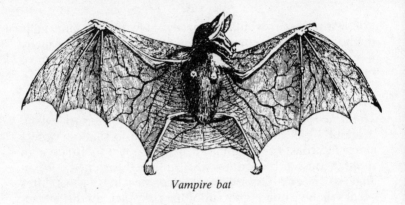

Vampire bat

at the earliest possible opportunity. Equally, it is important to institute supportive measures from the very outset, since many untreated patients will die before they reach the nearest hospital.

Animal bites (non-venomous)

Whenever the skin has been punctured by the teeth of a mammal, whether domestic or wild, referral to a physician is important. The greatest risk, other than haemorrhage and traumatic damage, is that of *rabies* (see also Section 3), followed by *tetanus*, and *septicaemia ('blood-poisoning')*. Rabies is not a risk, however, in Great Britain, Eire, Australia, New Zealand, Japan, Taiwan, Antarctica, or Scandinavia (including Iceland and Finland, but excluding Denmark). The main vectors (carriers) of rabies are foxes, skunks, domestic dogs and cats, and, in the Americas, Trinidad and Jamaica, bats (especially vampire bats, but also insectivorous or frugivorous species).

Following a bite, however minor, carry out the following measures *immediately*, and transport for medical advice:

(1) Clean the wound thoroughly with soap and running water for 5 minutes. Then irrigate thoroughly with 40% (or stronger) alcohol, such as gin or vodka.

(2) Control bleeding by pressure, and the internal administration of:

Arnica 30 ¼h

(3) Apply a *loose* dressing, and give *both* of the following internal remedies:

    (a) *Hydrophobinum 30 24h*
    (b) *Ledum 30 12h*

    [for convenience, alternate doses of *Ledum* may be given at the same time as the dose of *Hydrophobinum*]

In the absence of medical advice, these must be continued for at least *4 months*.

(4) Should wound infection occur, as witnessed by the presence of pus, continue with prescription (3), but give, in addition, both of the following internal remedies (they may be given together):

    (a) *Gunpowder 6 6h*
    (b) *Pyrogen 30 6h*

The infected wound itself should be cleaned with a mild antiseptic, such as *Rose Water (triple)* or *vinegar*. Loose wet dressings of the same may be applied.

Non-mammalian non-venomous bites, such as those from the crocodile, carry similar risks to those stated with regard to mammals, with the exception of rabies. Hence, they may be treated similarly, but the remedy *Hydrophobinum* may be excluded.

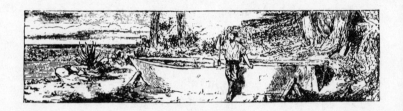

Some Diseases of The Skin

Heat, poor personal hygiene, and inadequate nutrition are conducive to skin disease. See also *Section 12* (for sunburn, prickly heat, etc.), *Section 17* (for foot problems), and *Section 22* (for ulcerative conditions).

Windburn and chaps
A cream may be applied to the skin several times daily, for both prevention and treatment, the formulation of which is as follows:

Cremoris Calendulae 5%	*30g*
d-Alpha Tocopheryl Acetati	*600IU*

Boil (Furuncle)
Boils are generally due to Staphylococcal bacteria. A discrete red and painful lump appears on the skin, which grows rapidly, becomes softer ('pointing'), and finally tends to discharge pus and dead material (termed 'the core'). Untreated, the whole process may take 3–14 days. They may be multiple. Boils affecting the outer ear canal are immensely painful. Sometimes the skin around the boil

becomes red and swollen. The administration of orthodox antibiotics is often worse than no treatment at all, since the condition may be perpetuated, rather than cured. Sometimes boils may be due to embedded foreign bodies (eg thorns, sea urchin spines), or secondary infection of insect bites. Occasionally, they may be a symptom of human *myiasis* (maggot infestation), the treatment of which is discussed later in this section. Care must be taken that the sufferer neither infects another, nor contaminates food or drink. Correction of hygiene and nutrition, and rest may be required. Persons suffering from recurrent boils should have the urine tested for glucose, since a small percentage will have diabetes mellitus (diabetes), which will require specialist treatment. A few others may have anaemia, the cause of which (eg hookworm disease, heavy periods) must be elucidated, and appropriate therapy given. The treatment of boils is as follows:

(1) Given early enough, the following internal remedy may induce speedy resolution without discharge, or given later, will hasten 'pointing':

Gunpowder 6 6h

(2) If the surrounding skin is swollen and hot, use the following internal remedy in conjunction with that stated in (1):

Belladonna 30 6h

(3) In addition to the above, where the boil is well developed, it may be encouraged to 'point' (soften), with subsequent discharge, by applying the following paste on clean dressings several times daily ('drawing a boil'):

Pasta Magnesii Sulphatis

(4) Where the boil is in the outer ear canal, the same paste should be applied liberally to a cotton tape, about 1.25cm × 5cm (½in × 2in), which should be gently teased with tweezers into the outer ear canal (but not pushed home tightly), allowing about 1.25cm (½in) to remain outside, for easy removal. This should be changed several times daily.

(5) Surgical incision is sometimes helpful, in order to hasten relief, but must only be carried out when the boil has 'pointed' (softened). In many cases, it may be avoided, by the measures given above.

(6) Where there is a low fever, the following may be taken internally, in conjunction with other measures:

> *Echinacea ø 5 drops 4h*
>
> [reduce the dose for children]

(7) Where boils are *recurrent*, without any obvious cause (eg diabetes, anaemia), the following internal remedy, given as *a single dose on three consecutive days*, may arrest the trait for some considerable time:

> *Anthracinum 200*

The following may be confused with simple boils:
(i) Infected sebaceous cyst (initial treatment similar to that given above).
(ii) Pestis minor (see Section 23).
(iii) Chagoma (see Section 26).
(iv) Trypanosomal chancre (see Section 26).
(v) Myiasis (see below).

Carbuncle
In reality, an extended boil (see above), with multiple discharging openings. The causation is similar. Treatment may be instituted along the same lines (see above), but the following internal remedy may be more effective than *Gunpowder*, for which it may be substituted:

> *Tarentula cubensis 30 6h*

A large number of botanic medicines have been used, mainly externally, in the treatment of boils and carbuncles. Proper advice with regard to their use should be sought. The following is a brief selection:

Allium spp. (wild onion). USA. Cheyenne Indians. Poultice of stems and bulbs applied. After discharge, irrigated with decoction of the same.
Aloe latifolia. South Africa. Leaf pulp applied.
Althaea officinalis (marshmallow). Poultice applied.

Anemone virginiana. USA. Menominee Indians. Pounded root poultice.

Avicennia officinalis. India. Green fruit poultice.

Betula lenta (black birch). USA. Tea from inner bark drunk.

Erythronium grandiflorum (glacier lily). USA. Blackfoot Indians. Pounded root as poultice.

Euphorbia brachyera (horned euphorbia). USA. Navajo Indians. Chewed plant applied.

Ficus carica (fig). Fresh fruit roasted, cut in half, and applied.

Lamium album (dead nettle). USA and Europe. Poultice of boiled leaves and flowers applied.

Linum lewisii (blue flax). USA. Paiute and Shoshoni Indians. Poultice applied.

Melilotus officinalis (yellow melilot). North America, Europe, Asia. Poultice applied.

Oberonia anceps. Indonesia. Crushed whole plant as poultice.

Pinus spp. (pine). USA. Choctaws. Pine gum, wax and fat applied.

Prunella vulgaris (common selfheal). USA. Quileute Indians. Poultice applied.

Rumex crispus (yellow dock). USA, Canada, Europe. Crushed leaves applied by North American Indians.

Ulmus fulva (slippery elm). USA. Potawatomis Indians. Bark used as poultice.

Zea mays (maize/corn). USA. Poultice of grain applied.

Cold sore (Herpes labialis)

Painful and tiny blisters (vesicles) of the lips, proceeding to scab formation. Cold sores are due to activation of a dormant Herpesvirus by sun, cold, stress, or the presence of another infection, such as the common cold (many people are especially prone to this condition, and homoeopathic constitutional treatment by an experienced practitioner can do much to reduce the trait). For their immediate treatment, take either of the following internal remedies:

(1) *Natrum muriaticum 30 6h*
(2) *Rhus toxicodendron 30 6h*

For *external* treatment, *surgical spirit* may be applied to early vesicles, every few hours. It is interesting to note that poultices of the bark of slippery elm (*Ulmus fulva*) were applied to cold sores by the Meskwaki Indians of the USA.

Impetigo
A highly contagious bacterial disease, usually of childhood, characterized by honey-coloured crusts overlying red areas of denuded skin. It usually is found on the face. It is important for the patient not to use another's towel, in order to prevent spread of infection. To treat, give either of the following remedies:

   (1) *Antimonium crudum 6 6h*
   (2) *Mezereum 6 6h*

Intertrigo (Inflammation of skin folds)
Increased sweating and poor hygiene in hot climates may lead to the development of soggy, weeping inflammation of skin-fold areas, such as between the buttocks, behind the ears, and beneath the breasts (especially if large and pendulous). Fungal infection is often present. See also *Dhobi's itch* (below). In addition to regular bathing, the following should be administered:

   (1) Externally a cream should be applied sparingly every 6 hours (*not* a greasy ointment), the formulation of which is as follows:

      Cremoris Graphitum 8x (D8)   30g
      Olei Melaleucae Alternifoliorum   10gtt

   (2) Additionally, the following internal remedy may be taken:

      Causticum 6 12h

Dhobi's itch (Washer[wo]man's itch/Tinea cruris)
A red, itchy, scaly rash of the upper parts of the inner thighs, and around the external genitalia, due to fungal infection in hot climates. A form of intertrigo (see above). Increased sweating, and poor hygiene are contributory. A similar condition may occur in the skin of the arm-pits (axillae). Excess-

ive scratching may lead to secondary bacterial infection, with the development of small or large boils (see above). In addition to regular bathing, treat as follows:

(1) A cream should be sparingly applied to the affected area every 6 hours, with the following formulation:

Unguenti Emulsificantis Aquosi	*30g*
Olei Melaleucae Alternifoliorum	*20gtt*
Violae Tricoloris ø	*5gtt*
Stellariae Mediae ø	*5gtt*

(2) Take internally:

Arsenicum iodatum 6 12h

Body Ringworm (Tinea circinata/Tinea corporis)

This is not a worm at all, but an extremely contagious fungal infection of the skin, very common in the tropics. Even in cool temperate climates, infection is not uncommon, where it may be contracted from contact with infected domestic pets, horses, cattle, or objects, such as fence posts, against which they have rubbed. In humans it is characterized by ring-shaped lesions, with slowly advancing, slightly raised, red and scaly borders, and central clearing. Some itching is experienced. The microscopy of skin scrapings will help to confirm the diagnosis, where such is available. A more severe variety, *tinea imbricata (Tokelau ringworm)*, chiefly found in the South Pacific islands and Eastern Archipelago, is characterized by multiple concentric circular lesions, and is due to a specific species of fungus. Body ringworm may be treated as follows:

(1) A cream, of the following formulation, should be applied every 12 hours (remember to wash your hands after use, to prevent the spread of infection elsewhere, or to others):

Unguenti Emulsificantis Aquosi	*30g*
Olei Melaleucae Alternifoliorum	*20gtt*
Hydrastidis ø	*10gtt*

(2) In addition, the following internal remedy may be taken:

Tellurium 6 12h

In resistant cases, the homoeopathic remedy Bacillinum, given high and infrequently, will often assist, with regard to ringworm of either scalp or body. It should be given under the supervision of an homoeopathic practitioner, and is not recommended during pregnancy.

Scalp ringworm (Tinea capitis)

This fungal infection of the scalp is almost exclusively seen in children, and tends to disappear spontaneously at puberty. It resembles ringworm of cattle. Round, grey, scaly patches appear on the scalp, apparently bald. In actuality, the hairs of the patch are broken off where they emerge from the skin. There may be slight itching. Treatment should include:

(1) External treatment of 'bald' patches twice daily with the cream suggested for *body ringworm (see above)*.

(2) *External* application of the following formulation to the remaining scalp and hair, *20–40 drops once daily*:

Olei Olivae	9ml
Olei Melaleucae Alternifoliorum	1ml

(3) Internally, give:

Dulcamara 6 12h

See note above concerning the use of Bacillinum

Numerous botanic treatments have been applied externally for the treatment of both body and scalp ringworm. It may be of interest to note some of them:

Adenia singaporeana. Malaya. Root decoction.
Aloe latifolia. South Africa. Leaf pulp and juice.
Aloe saponaria. ditto
Arum maculatum. Ointment of plant.
Asclepias exalta. USA. Rappahannock Indians. Latex.
Betula nigra. USA. Catawba Indians. Boiled buds plus sulphur.
Bulbine asphodeloides. South Africa. Leaf and stalk juice.
Bulbine narcissifolia. ditto
Cassia occidentalis. Tropics. Seeds.
Cassia sophera. Tropics. Leaf juice.
Cassia tora. India. Leaves.

Chelidonium majus. USA/Europe. Ointment/poultice of plant.
Ipomoea pandurata. USA. Root.
Juglans nigra. USA. Poultice of green fruit rind.
Leea macrophylla. India. Root.
Lobelia inflata. USA. Plant poultice.
Microstemon velutina. South-East Asia. Bark latex.
Morus spp. USA. Rappahannock Indians. Leaf axis latex.
Pentaspadon motleyi. Malayan Archipelago. Stem balsam.
Plantago major. North America/Europe. Plant decoction.
Rhinacanthus nasutas. India. Fresh roots/leaves/seeds plus lime juice.
Sanguinaria canadensis. USA. Iroquois Indians. Root.
Smilax officinalis. USA. Plant infusion.

Pityriasis versicolor (Tinea versicolor)

A fungal infection of the skin, commoner in those who sweat a great deal, and commonly seen in the tropics. Whilst it is not particularly contagious, epidemics may occur amongst athletes. The lesions vary from 4mm in diameter to large confluent areas. In dark-skinned people the lesions are usually paler than the surrounding skin, and generally fawn in colour, although in one variety of this disease, pityriasis versicolor alba, they are frankly white. In light-skinned races they may be darker than the surrounding skin, or appear as areas that fail to tan properly. There may be mild itching. Microscopy of skin scrapings, when available, assists in confirmation of the diagnosis. The treatment will differ for the hypopigmented (pale patches) and hyperpigmented (dark patches) types of this disorder:

(1) Hyperpigmented type:
(a) Apply the following cream *every 12 hours*:

Unguenti Emulsificantis Aquosi	30g
Olei Melaleucae Alternifoliorum	15gtt
Sepiae 3x(D3)	1gt

(b) Additionally, take internally:

Sepia 6 12h

189

(2) Hypopigmented type:
(a) Apply the following cream *every 12 hours*:

Unguenti Emulsificantis Aquosi	*30g*
Olei Melaleucae Alternifoliorum	*15gtt*
Ammi Majoris ø	*10gtt*
Olei Bergamottae	*5gtt*

(b) Additionally, take this mixed remedy internally *12h*:
Ammi majus 3x(D3)
Tellurium 6

[exposure to sunlight is also necessary for repigmentation to occur]

Notes

(i) The remedy Bacillinum may be useful in resistant cases. See above, under 'body ringworm', for details.

(ii) Pityriasis versicolor, especially the alba type, must be differentiated from vitiligo, a non-fungal depigmentation of the skin, which is difficult to treat. Whilst pityriasis versicolor mainly involves the trunk (although lesions on arms, thighs, neck, and face can occur), vitiligo mainly presents with lesions around the orifices, or on the finger tips. Moreover, itching does not occur with vitiligo. Obviously, microscopy is also helpful.

Otomycosis (Panama ear/Surfer's ear/Hot weather ear)

This unpleasant condition, common in white people visiting tropical or subtropical climates, is due to fungal infection of the outer ear canal, sometimes with additional bacterial elements. Whilst swimming may aggravate the disorder, the wearing of ear-plugs is not protective against it. Initially, the outer ear canal becomes sore, with considerable itching, and pain on touch or when chewing. The pain increases, becoming worse at night, and the itching may become intolerable. A mild fever may develop in severe cases. Considerable amounts of debris accumulate in the outer ear canal, and the lining becomes swollen, leading to deafness, which is reversible with appropriate therapy. Treatment may be given as follows:

(1) The following formulation should be instilled into the ear, *5–10 drops 6h* [shake well before use]:

Aquae Rosae (Triplicis)	*5ml*
Spiritus (90%)	*5ml*
Olei Melaleucae Alternifoliorum	*10gtt*

(2) In advanced cases, with the accumulation of much debris, it is desirable to treat the ear with *hydrogen peroxide* solution immediately before each instillation of the above drops. The solution must be freshly prepared each time, in the proportion of 2 drops of hydrogen peroxide (3%/10 volume) to 3 drops of clean water. *5–10 drops* of this dilution should be instilled into the ear, allowing it to act for about 5 minutes; thereafter wiping out any debris or fluid with cotton-wool buds. The formulation given in (1) may then be instilled. The undiluted hydrogen peroxide must be stored in dark, well-sealed bottles, away from daylight, and preferably in a cool place.

(3) Additionally, take internally:

Mercurius solubilis 6 6h

[in lesser cases, *Silicea 6, Pulsatilla 6, or Hepar sulphuris 6* may be usefully substituted]

Scabies (Burrowing mite infestation)

A parasitic disease of the skin caused by the mite *Sarcoptes scabiei*, which burrows into the skin, and is barely visible to the naked eye. Of world-wide distribution, it is acquired by close contact with an infested individual, or sleeping in their bedding. Except in infants, the infestation generally spares the head and neck. There is severe itching, worse at night. The lesions consist of little blisters (vesicles), pustules (pus-filled vesicles), and raised itchy lumps (papules). Along the sides of the fingers and the heels of the palms, 'runs' may be seen in the form of short, irregular, linear marks, about 2–3mm long. Microscopy of the skin, when available, confirms the diagnosis. It may be treated as follows:

(1) Launder all clothing and bedding.
(2) Take the following internal remedy:

Sulphur 6 12h

[avoid the use of higher potencies]

(3) Additionally, apply the following ointment to affected areas *once a week*:

Balsami Peruviani	*12.5%*
Unguenti Simplicis	*87.5%*

[this may cause dermatitis in sensitive individuals]

Pediculosis (Louse infestation)

Human louse infestation is to be found in three main forms, each caused by a separate variety of this insect: pediculosis corporis (of the body), pediculosis capitis (of the scalp), and pediculosis pubis (of the pubic region). They are largely diseases of poor hygiene and overcrowding. Pediculosis pubis ('crabs') is, however, usually spread by sexual relations, although it may be acquired from an infested toilet seat. The communal use of combs and headwear facilitates the dissemination of pediculosis capitis. All three types are associated with reactions consequent upon the bites of these lice. There is often severe itching, and scratching leads to gross excoriation of the skin, sometimes with secondary infection, and the appearance of small pus-filled blisters (pustules). The body louse, some 3–4mm long, is seldom to be discovered on the skin, upon which it merely feeds, but in the seams of clothing, where it may be found upon careful examination, along with its eggs ('nits'). Rarely, nits of body lice may be found attached to the fine body hair of children. The pubic louse is smaller, and its presence is usually inferred by an intense skin reaction. Its nits are attached to the shafts of the pubic hair. Occasionally it attacks other areas, such as the eyelashes or moustache. Head lice are most easily identified by their pale nits, which, unlike dandruff, are firmly attached to the hair. They are most easily identified on the hair of the nape of the neck, or that above the ears. In severe cases, the hair is matted together with a solidified purulent material, stemming from an intense reaction to the bites. Only the body louse is significant with regard to the transmission of major disease, such as typhus and relapsing fever. Treatment must include: killing the lice, removing the nits, and reducing the skin reaction. To these ends, the following may be found helpful:

(1) Body lice are simply eradicated by careful laundering of clothes. In children, however, the fine body hair (vellus hair) should be inspected for nits, and the affected hair shaved off with a razor.

(2) Head and pubic lice may be killed with any one of the following three homoeopathic preparations:

    (a) *Staphysagria ø*
    (b) *Quassia ø*
    (c) **Sabadilla ø*

    *[doctor's prescription required in UK]

Whichever is chosen, 2–3ml should be rubbed well into the hair and skin *once daily*. If the skin is not too sensitive, as with early infestations, the undiluted form may be used. Where the skin is broken, however, from scratching or dermatitis, the mother tincture should be diluted with an equal volume of clean water before application. It is preferable to shampoo and dry the hair before applying the homoeopathic preparation. A fine-toothed comb, known as a *nit comb*, should be used twice daily to remove adherent nits. If such is unavailable, the hair must be shaved close to the skin.

(3) Treatment for skin reaction may include:

    (a) The external application of the following cream 6h:

Cremoris Graphitum 8x(D8)	*30g*
Stellariae Mediae ø	*10 gtt*
Ledi ø	*10gtt*

    (b) In general, the following alternation of internal remedies:

Sulphur 6 morning and evening
Ledum 6 at midday

[avoid the use of higher potencies]

    (c) Where the scalp is badly affected, with much

purulent discharge, the hair should be cut off, and the following internal remedy given in preference to the former prescription:

Mezereum 6 6h

Myiasis (Human maggot infestation)

This is the name given for the presence of fly *maggots* within the tissues or organs of the body. There are three main types:

(1) *Specific*. Caused by species, such as the Congo floor maggot, human botfly and tumbu fly, which are confirmed parasites, and are obliged to be so. These are discussed in detail below.

(2) *Semispecific*. Caused by species which may either develop in human tissue or in external organic matter, such as food. These mainly infest open wounds, and usually attack only dying or dead tissue. Indeed, under primitive circumstances, with no surgical help available, the presence of these maggots, whilst unaesthetic, may be most desirable from the therapeutic point of view. In former times, the introduction of the maggot of the black bottle fly was efficacious in the treatment of osteomyelitis (inflammation and death of bone tissue). In modern times, however, we would be more inclined to remove the 'offending' maggots, and treat otherwise. Most of the flies responsible for this condition are distributed worldwide, with the exception of the common screw worm fly (western hemisphere only). They include: green bottle, blue bottle, black bottle, flesh fly, stable fly, non-biting stable fly, and housefly.

(3) *Accidental*. Caused by species which can occasionally adapt to life within the intestine, or urinary and genital passages. The most common maggots causing intestinal myiasis are those of the latrine fly and lesser housefly. Infestation is acquired by eating or drinking fly eggs or maggots, or by flies depositing eggs or maggots on the anus during defecation. Symptoms are variable, and include: lack of appetite, abdominal pain, nausea, vomiting, diarrhoea, and black stools (melaena). In the 18th Century in England, Stilton cheese was often eaten riddled with maggots, and a 'maggot

spoon' provided for their consumption, or, at least, so it is said. Sometimes the maggots are readily visible in the motions. Treatment with purgatives is often efficacious. *Oleum Ricini* (castor oil), given in milk or fruit juice as a single dose of *10–20ml* for adults (*5–10ml* for children 5–12 years of age), should suffice. Infestation of the urinary or genital tract is relatively rare, and is due to either the migration of maggots from the intestinal tract (via the anus), or the deposition of eggs or maggots by flies upon the genital aperture (especially of females). Symptoms resembling cystitis (such as burning, frequency, blood in the urine) occur, plus the spontaneous passage of maggots. Surgical removal is necessary.

Let us now return to 'specific' myiasis, that type caused by obligate parasitic maggots, and consider the different varieties in detail, with regard to geographical distribution, avoidance and therapy. You will observe that 'boils' ('furuncles') and deep purulent wounds are a fairly common feature of infestation, and in these cases, along with any other therapeutic measures suggested, the use of the internal remedy *Gunpowder 6 6h* is to be recommended:

(a) *Congo floor maggot*. Tropical Africa. The maggot hides in the ground during the day, and bores into the skin to suck blood at night, leaving a small hole. It is, therefore, only found on the host at night. Avoid sleeping on the ground, especially on the floors of native huts. Eggs and maggots are transported by sleeping mats of itinerants. The use of repellents on both skin and bedding is advisable (see *Section 14*).

(b) *Tumbu fly*. Tropical Africa. Young maggots invade unbroken skin, producing often multiple 'boils'. Two black dots, the breathing apparatus of the maggot (spiracles), are often visible at the surface of the boil. Mineral oil or water should be applied to these, and the boil gently squeezed to extrude the maggot, which may be some 12–15mm long when fully developed. Even without treatment the fully developed maggot will quit its host after 8–9 days. The female fly deposits her eggs in polluted soil, or clothing, especially if it smells of sweat or urine. Clothes hung out to

195

dry, or left on the ground are prime targets. Hot ironing destroys the eggs. Avoid drying clothes outdoors. Avoid sleeping on polluted ground.

(c) *Human botfly*. Mexico, Central America, tropical South America, and especially the forested eastern slopes of the Andes. The fly glues its eggs to mosquitoes or other carriers, such as ticks and biting flies, which then convey them to the human skin, most commonly the exposed areas. The lesion produced is a 'boil', rather like that produced by the Tumbu fly maggot (see above), which becomes intensely painful. Similarly, the respiratory spiracles may be visible. There is, however, considerable local destruction of tissue, and the maggots will not leave the tissues spontaneously until 50–100 days have passed, when full development has been reached. Native Indians incise the 'boil', apply *tobacco juice*, and then squeeze out the maggot. Avoidance of mosquito, fly, and tick bites is most important, in view of the mode of transmission of this disease (see *Section 14*).

(d) *Flesh flies*. Western USA, Mediterranean, near East, former USSR. According to species, there may be invasion of unbroken skin, wounds, nose, or ears. One species produces disfiguring wounds, others produce 'boils' (see above). Babies are prime targets, where the neck is a favourite site of attack. Maggots should be physically removed. Again, insect repellent techniques are important for prevention, as they are for the other forms of specific myiasis described below (see *Section 14*).

(e) *Primary screw worm fly*. Southern USA, American tropics. Maggots may invade wounds, sinuses, ears, or nose, the latter being the commonest site of attack. Deep, purulent and malodorous wounds are characteristic, with erosion of bone. The mortality rate is about 8%. The maggots must be physically removed. In screw worm country, all persons who wish to sleep in the day should be protected with bed nets. Persons who have wounds, nasal catarrh, or eye discharge, are particularly attractive to the fly. Blood-stained bandages or clothes also serve as a lure.

(f) *Old World screw worm fly*. Orient, Ethiopia. Similar in many respect to primary screw worm disease, but lesions may occur virtually anywhere, including the eye. Prevention and treatment are similar.

(g) Less frequent causes of specific myiasis are the horse botfly, cattle warble flies, sheep botflies, rodent botfly, and the head botfly of horses.

Creeping eruption (Cutaneous larva migrans/ Sandworm)

This condition, also known as 'plumber's' or 'duckhunter's itch', is usually due to infection with the larvae of the cat or dog *hookworm*. Creeping eruption occurs in most humid tropical and subtropical climates, and is particularly contracted in the USA, along the coast of the Gulf of Mexico and Florida, and along the coasts of Sri Lanka, South, East and West Africa. It is not uncommon in the Caribbean, coastal South America, and Thailand. Summer and early autumn (fall) are associated with more infections. The disease is generally contracted by walking in bare feet on sandy beaches *above the high-water mark*, which can usually be recognised as the highest line of washed-up debris. It can also be contracted by crawling under beach huts (hence, 'plumber's itch'), and from skin contact with the mounds of nutria and racoons in marshes (hence, 'duckhunter's itch'). Most lesions are found on the feet and hands, but their characteristics are similar at all sites. The animal hookworm, incapable of invasion into deeper tissues, remains within the bounds of the skin to produce slowly moving (several millimetres per day), hardened, sinuous red lines, accompanied by much itching, and sometimes blistering. A similar condition may arise from infection with non-human strains of the worm *Strongyloides*, acquired by skin contact with contaminated mounds in tropical swamps, and for which the treatment is similar. Therapy may be given along these lines:

(1) Externally, apply the following cream to the affected area *6h*:

Unguenti Emulsificantis Aquosi	*30g*
Olei Chenopodii	*10gtt*
Olei Thymi	*10gtt*

(2) Additionally, take the following internal remedy:

Sulphur 6 6h

(3) An alternative to those measures given above is to freeze the advancing head of the red track with an *ethyl chloride* spray.

Differential diagnosis

There are several important conditions which resemble creeping eruption, but for which the treatment is different. Medical expertise should be sought, where possible:

(1) Human Strongyloides (nematode) infection [strongyloidiasis]. From skin contact (especially bare feet) with moist village soil in tropics and subtropics. It may coexist in the same individual with hookworm (see Section 27). Itchy, rapidly moving, serpentine, non-hardened red lines and weals (restricted to area between knees and neck), persisting for a few hours at a time [termed 'larva currens']. Most established infections are, however, without symptoms. Early infection may be associated with cough, wheeze, upper abdominal pain, fatty diarrhoea, and weight loss.

(2) Gnathostoma (nematode) infection [gnathostomiasis]. Infection acquired by eating inadequately cooked fish. Commonest in Thailand. Also Vietnam, Malaya, India, Japan. Migrating tracks of skin swelling, lasting 7–10 days, and recurring every 2–6 weeks.

(3) Paragonimus (fluke) infection [paragonimiasis]. Mostly contracted by eating raw or undercooked crabs. Also accidental transfer to the mouth when preparing raw crabs for cooking. Japan (crab soup), Philippines ('kinagang'), Korea (raw crab), China ('drunken crab'). Migrating nodules under skin in children are a sign of this disease in China and Thailand.

(4) Sparganosis (tapeworm infection). Mainly Japan, Korea, China, Vietnam, Indonesia, Central Africa (Masai). Occasionally, Europe (Holland), South America, USA. Accidental drinking of contaminated water. Ingestion of raw flesh of snakes, mammals, or frogs. Rubbing raw split frogs on eye or skin diseases (China). Swollen and intensely painful skin lesions, which may resemble acne, with pustular nodules.

(5) Myiasis (see above). Migrating maggots.

Swimmer's itch (Cercarial dermatitis/Clam digger's itch)

This skin condition arises from penetration of the skin by the cercariae (immature forms) of certain *schistosomes* (blood flukes) which only produce serious disease in animals or birds. Having penetrated the human skin, *they die*. They do, however, cause a localised skin reaction, the nature of which is dependent upon the sensitivity of the subject. An intensely itchy, lumpy red rash appears, which, in many instances, disappears within a day or so. In those who have previously been sensitized, the rash may persist for 7–10 days, and will be more of the nature of a florid dermatitis. The disease is mainly one of fresh water, but has been reported in brackish and coastal waters of the USA, in the Atlantic seaboard, Gulf Coast, California and Hawaii. The disease is endemic in Canada, Wisconsin, Michigan, and Minnesota. In Colorado it occurs up to 2750m (9000ft). It has been found in Argentina, El Salvador, Colombia, and Mexico. Outbreaks have occurred in Holland, Wales, Switzerland, Germany, France, Malaya, Japan, Africa, and New Zealand. The intermediate hosts for the parasite are various species of water snail. Since the disorder is self-limiting and relatively benign, the primary aim of treatment is to improve the comfort of the patient:

(1) Apply the following lotion *externally*, every hour or two:

Cupri Sulphatis	*5g*
Caerulei Methyleni	*2g*
Aquae	*ad 100ml*

(2) Additionally, the following internal remedy may be taken:

Antimonium tartaricum 6 6h

Warning!: A similar condition to swimmer's itch may be produced by human varieties of schistosome, which cause the important disease *bilharziasis*. Here, the immature blood flukes tend to survive, further invading the tissues of the body, and causing serious disease. The geographical distribution, clinical features, prevention, and treatment of this disease are discussed in detail in *Section 21*. Any person contracting what appears to be swimmer's itch in a bilharziasis zone should receive urgent treatment along the lines stated in that section.

Urticating caterpillar hairs
Several groups of caterpillars bear hairs, associated with poison secreting cells, which are capable of producing irri-

tation to the skin or eyes. Either direct contact with the caterpillar, or contact with moulted hairs blown by the wind will produce a reaction. Hairs may be found on washing hung out to dry. Epidemics of this disorder are not infrequent, and one recently occurred on the southern coast of England, Portland Bill in Dorset being one of the worst affected areas. The caterpillars of the *browntail moth* were the offenders in this instance. The rash produced by these larvae is intensely itchy, and resembles rubella (German measles). The lesions are slightly raised, red or pink in colour, sometimes with an orange tint in the centre. Spontaneous resolution may take up to 7 days. Treat internally with:

Pulsatilla 6 6h

In the USA, the *puss caterpillar (Megalopyge opercularis)* is certainly the most important offending species. In Texas, schools have been closed on occasions, due to its presence on playgrounds. The initial symptom produced is an intense burning pain, spreading rapidly beyond the contact site, and lasting as long as 12 hours. The affected area develops white bumps (papules) which soon turn red, and local swelling occurs. There may be nausea, fever, and local numbness. Paralysis may occur, particularly if contact is received on the neck area. Severe symptoms can persist for about 6 days. Treatment may be given as follows:

(1) External application of warm *dilute ammonia water (Liquor Ammoniae Dil.)*, or a paste of *baking soda* and water.

(2) Additionally, the internal administration of:

Sulphur 6 2h

(3) Additionally, the following internal remedy, if available, may be given in conjunction with (2):

Megalopygis opercularis larva 30 2h

Blister beetles

Certain beetles contain within their bodies toxic substances, which are released when the insects are crushed, leading to blistering of the skin. In Europe, the best known is the

Spanish fly. Other varieties occur in the USA, where they are most problematical between July and September (especially for potato workers), in Java, South America, certain Pacific islands (coconut beetles), and tropical South and East Africa. Some species are associated with delayed blistering, which may take 1–2 days to appear. The blisters may be quite large (bullae), and secondary infection may occur, if inadequately protected. The affected area should be washed with a solution of *bicarbonate of soda* before a dressing is applied. Internal treatment may be given with:

Cantharis 30 6h

A different type of irritation is produced by the *small flour beetle* which gives off a gaseous irritant, affecting the eyes and nose.

Shellfish urticaria (hives/nettle-rash)
A raised and itchy rash produced by allergy to fish or shellfish. Usually the allergy is specific to one or several varieties of fish or shellfish, and only occasionally is more general. Further ingestion of the appropriate items is obviously best avoided, unless some form of homoeopathic desensitization can be instituted. The rash itself may be treated internally with:

Urtica urens 6 2h

Toxicodendron dermatitis (Poison ivy rash/Rhus dermatitis)
Plants of the genus *Toxicodendron* are an important cause of dermatitis in North America. All parts of these plants are capable of producing an allergic skin reaction, including the roots. It is said that even the smoke produced by burning them will produce the same response. The plants involved are:

(a) *Poison ivy (Toxicodendron radicans/Rhus toxicodendron)*. Commonly found in the river valleys of North America. Homoeopathic potencies (dilutions) of this plant are commonly used in the treatment of certain rheumatic complaints.

(b) *Poison oak (Toxicodendron diversilobum and Toxico-dendron quercifolium)*. Common on the West Coast.
(c) *Poison sumac (Toxicodendron vernix)*. Common everywhere in the USA, except the West Coast.

These plants are either climbing vines, or crawling species, with three clustered leaflets, green and waxy in the spring, and yellow or red, with white berries, in the autumn (fall). An oily resin known as *toxicodendrol* is present in all species, which contains the active allergenic substance *urushiol*. Even the slightest contact with these plants may induce a rash. Only a very few are immune to its action. Initial exposure results in a rash some 9–14 days later, whilst subsequent contact induces a rash within a few hours or days. The rash consists of groups of small blisters (vesicles), resembling herpes simplex (see *cold sores*, above), or large blisters (bul-lae). It is intensely itchy and painful, with a red base, and tends to weep. *If the skin is washed thoroughly within 10 minutes of contact, the rash can be prevented.* Toxicodendron dermatitis is notorious for the ease with which it can be spread to other parts of the skin. The smallest amount of toxicodendrol under the finger nails or on the clothing may cause contact reactions to occur elsewhere. Once the rash is acquired, it is a good idea to wash the affected part with a good volume of flowing water, scrub hands and fingernails, shower, and change and launder all clothing. Treatment of the established rash may be given as follows:

(1) Give either of the following internal remedies:
  (a) *Ledum 30 6h*
  (b) *Rhus toxicodendron 30 6h*
(2) Additionally, apply the following lotion externally *2h*:

Grindelia ø 1 drop + water 9 drops

This use of *Grindelia* (gum plant) is derived from the botanic medicine of the Indian tribes of northern California. As might be expected, the North American Indians used a number of other plants for the external treatment of this disorder:
Artemisia spp. (wormwood). Yokias. ?parts of plant used.

Astragalus nitidus and Astragalus succulentus (milk vetch). Cheyennes. Leaves and stems (presumably dry) ground to fine powder and sprinkled on weeping lesions.

Comptonia peregrina (sweet fern). Mohegans. Leaves steeped in water.

Impatiens biflora (jewelweed/touch-me-not). Potawatomis. Juice applied. Recent experiences with a freezable decoction of this plant have tended to confirm its efficacy.

Lactuca canadensis (wild lettuce). Menominees. Juice of freshly picked leaves applied.

Yucca glauca and Chlorogalum pomeridianum (soaproot). Pomos. Lotion of soapy juice applied.

Gympie Gympie dermatitis (Stinging tree rash)

The larger leaves of the gympie gympie tree of the tropical rain forests of Australia possess hairs, which induce an extremely painful rash, accompanied by swelling. Fortunately, thanks to the benevolence of Nature, a plant grows in its immediate vicinity, the juice of which, when applied, is a powerful antidote to its effects. This is the *cunjeboy*, a type of lily.

Manchineel dermatitis

See Section 11, under 'Manchineel poisoning'

Nettle stings

Whilst the experience might be painful, it is usually brief. It is interesting to note that there are recorded instances of the *temporary* alleviation of rheumatic conditions in those who have fallen into beds of nettles (bee stings have also produced a similar result on odd occasions). Relief from nettle stings may be obtained by rubbing with a dock leaf, rhubarb leaf, or the juice of the stem of the nettle itself. The application of the juice of a common land snail, whilst probably effective, would seem somewhat unappealing.

Algae dermatitis

Contact with certain types of blue-green algae can produce a reaction in the skin of swimmers. This has been reported along the coast of Hawaii and elsewhere. The rash resembles that of *Toxicodendron dermatitis* (see above), but is less severe, and resolves fairly quickly. It may be treated internally with:

Rhus toxicodendron 30 6h

Tropical wood dermatitis

Allergy to tropical hard and soft woods is not uncommon in those who work with them, such as loggers, carpenters, and picture framers. The important varieties of wood in this respect are Iroko (African teak), Obeche (wa-wa), satin wood, teak, and mahogany. Reactions may vary from a simple irritating contact dermatitis of the hands, to facial swelling, accompanied by symptoms resembling hay-fever. Subsequent exposure to the wood or sawdust may lead to progressive worsening of the condition. Once aware of the probable cause of the problem, avoidance is obviously the most expedient course of action. For those, however, who must continue working with these materials, some success in prevention may be procured by taking an homoeopathic remedy made from the offending wood itself. This should be taken from at least a few hours prior to exposure, and continued until a few days after the event. By way of example:

Obeche 6 12h

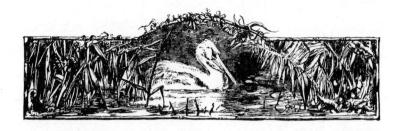

Section 17

SOME DISORDERS OF LEGS AND FEET

See also *Section 5* (travel swelling), *Section 11* (gout), *Section 12* (heat effects), *Section 13* (chilblains, frostbite), *Section 18* (fracture), and *Section 22* (ulcers).

Tired and aching feet (Podalgia)
From prolonged exercise, or standing:

    (1) *Scilla maritima 6 2h*
    (2) *Arnica 30 2h*

Tired leg muscles
From exercise:

       Arnica 30 2h

Bruised feet
From walking on hard ground, pebbles, or rocks, especially in bare feet:

       Arnica 30 2h

Corn (Clavus)
Apply the following cream *12h*:

Cremor Calendulae 5%

Ingrowing toenail
Often a result of excessive cutting of the corners of the great toenail. In addition to seeking the advice of a chiropodist (podiatrist), consider:

Magnetis polus Australis 30 12h

Cracked heels with hard skin
Often aggravated by ill-fitting shoes or 'flip-flops', and taking showers rather than baths. In addition to using a pumice stone after bathing:

Antimonium crudum 6 12h

Blistered feet
From ill-fitting shoes, running, or walking:

(1) Clean the foot with soap and water. Puncture the blister with a needle sterilized in a flame. Express the liquid (serum).

(2) Thereafter, apply the following cream on a clean dressing, renewing it *6–12h*:

Cremor Calendulae 5%

Nocturnal calf cramps
These may be a symptom of inadequate salt intake (see *Section 12*), or back problems, for which the services of a chiropractor or osteopath should be sought, especially if such a practitioner includes *sterile* acupuncture in his skills. Established calf cramp requires urgent mechanical treatment: grasp all the toes of the affected side firmly, and bend them back sharply towards the top of the foot. Repeat this manoeuvre several times. To prevent night cramps, should an increase in salt intake fail, consider:

Cuprum metallicum 30, one dose 30 minutes before retiring

Swimmer's cramp

For treatment:

Cuprum metallicum 30 every 10 minutes

For prevention:

Cuprum metallicum 30 6h

Burning foot syndrome

A frequently undiagnosed cause of burning pain in the feet is *pantothenic acid deficiency*. The following should be taken for several months:

Calcium pantothenate 500mg 12h

[adult dose]

Metatarsalgia

Pain in the ball of the foot, or on the top of the foot, immediately behind the toes. This is often due to minor dislocation of the toes, leading to excessive pressure on the heads of the metatarsal bones (long bones) of the foot. Treatment is largely mechanical, and is more easily achieved when administered by another person. Grasp each toe firmly by its base, with the thumb pressing down on the top of the latter. Pull out sharply in line with the long axis of the foot. The toe will then snap into a correct position. This procedure, which takes a little practice, should be repeated daily. Additionally, if the heads of the metatarsals are significantly tender, that is to say bruised, take the following internal remedy:

Ruta graveolens 6 6h

Sprain

This is damage to the ligaments of a joint. Ankle and knee sprains are not uncommon, and are often accompanied by much pain and swelling. If the disability is severe, there may be confusion with a fracture. Sprains may be treated as follows:

(1) Apply ice (bags of frozen vegetables may be used), or cold water compresses, to reduce the swelling. The efficacy of the cold water compress will be increased by the

addition of 5ml (1 teaspoon) of *Arnica ø* to every 500ml (1 pint) of water.

(2) Internally, *Arnica 30* should be given, initially every half hour for several hours, then hourly, reducing the frequency to once every 4 hours, as improvement occurs. *Ledum 30*, may be given instead with similar frequency in the case of ankle sprains, for which it may be marginally better than *Arnica*.

(3) Once the swelling has started to reduce, a crepe bandage may be applied to support the injured ligament. In the case of a sprained *ankle*, the bandage should be applied from behind the toes to just below the knee, firmly but not tightly. In the case of a twisted *knee*, localised bandaging of the knee is *not recommended*, since there is a risk of producing clots in the deep veins of the calf muscles, which may pass to the lungs, with possible fatal consequences (pulmonary embolism). In order to support a knee, the crepe bandage should be applied, firmly but not tightly, from just above the ankle to just above the knee (lower thigh).

(4) Should there be some persistence of symptoms after 7 days, *Arnica* may be stopped, and the following remedy given:

> *Strontium carbonicum 30 12h*

Pulled muscle

A common cause of acute calf pain in athletic persons. Give:

(1) Severe pain, incapable of all movement:

> *Bryonia 30 ½h*

(2) Subsequently, instead of the above:

> *Agaricus muscarius 6 6h*

Athlete's foot (Tinea pedis)

A soggy, peeling condition occurring between the toes, due to fungal infection. It is encouraged by poor hygiene, hot climates, nylon socks, and soles and uppers of man-made materials. Open shoes, where possible, canvas shoes or boots, and cotton socks are recommended. Treat as follows:

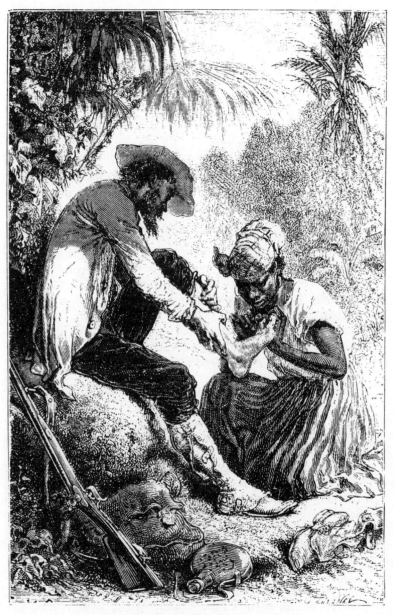

Maria extracting chegoes from John's feet

(1) Apply the following cream 2–3 times daily:
   Unguenti Emulsificantis Aquosi   *30g*
   Olei Melaleucae Alternifoliorum   *20gtt*

(2) Additionally, take internally:

   Graphites 6 6h

Verruca (Plantar wart)

A localised area of hard skin, due to infection with a wart virus. Often acquired from swimming pools or communal showers, it is only transmissible to susceptible individuals. Verrucae may be found on the undersurfaces of the toes or feet, around the heels, and occasionally on the finger tips. They may be differentiated from simple hard skin by the presence of a characteristic black dot or tiny hole at the centre, and the extreme tenderness that is elicited on pressure. A verruca is usually several millimetres in diameter, but may be considerably larger. Some success in treating verrucae has been procured by applying *black (over-ripe) banana skin* under an occlusive plaster. An alternative method, which I might say has been highly effective in virtually all cases I have treated myself, is as follows:

(1) Take a shower, bath or foot-bath each day. Immediately after, abrade the verruca with a pumice stone.
(2) Sterilize a thick sewing needle in a flame. Apply a drop of *Thuja* ø to the verruca with a small wooden stick (such as a matchstick). Do not worry if it contacts normal skin, since it is completely non-corrosive (it is *poisonous* if taken internally). With the sharp end of the needle held at about 30° to the surface of the skin, apply firm pressure, and scratch the liquid into the surface of the verruca in the manner of cross-hatching. Do not draw blood. Repeat the process of liquid application and scratching several times, until the verruca is light brown in colour. Resterilize the needle.
(3) This technique should be carried out on a daily basis, where possible. It kills the wart virus, with consequent reduction of tenderness, and final expulsion of the core of

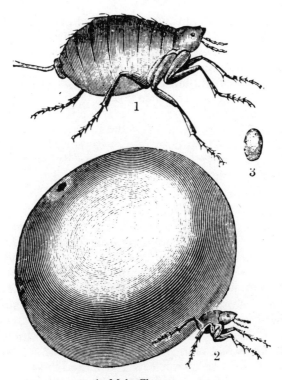

1. Male Chego.
2. Female Chego, dilated with eggs.
3. Egg.

the verruca. In stubborn cases, it may be necessary to continue treatment for up to 6 weeks.

Jiggers (Chigoes/Chegoes)

These are the pregnant females of the sand flea, *Tunga pene-trans*, found extensively in the tropical areas of the Americas and Africa. They are also to be found on the West coast of India. The fertilized jigger burrows into the skin of her victim, usually around a toenail, but sometimes between the toes, or on the sole of the foot, and occasionally elsewhere. After 8–12 days, an irritating and painful swelling appears, caused by the distention of the flea with eggs. The lesions

211

may be single, or multiple. Complications include: ulceration, secondary infection with pus formation, tetanus, and gas gangrene. Obviously, this is yet another reason to avoid walking in bare feet in tropical areas.

The condition should be treated by 'surgical' removal of the flea. Enlarge the entrance hole of the jigger with a sterile needle (the needle may be sterilized in a flame). Apply gentle pressure to the sides of the lesion, in order to expel the flea intact. Clean the wound with an antiseptic, such as *Rose Water (triple)*, and apply a loose dressing, saturated with same.

Mycetoma (Madura foot/Maduromycosis)

This disease is not contagious, but is due to fungal infection acquired by traumatic implantation, especially via thorns (from acacias in particular) or splinters. It generally involves feet or hands, but may involve the skull. In the foot (madura foot) it often begins as a painless nodule on the sole of the foot. The fungus then slowly invades the deeper tissues forming multiple abscesses, with progressive enlargement of the foot over a period of years. After some time (up to 6 years), sinuses (channels to the skin surface) appear, which discharge pus and characteristic coloured grains of fungus. A variety of different fungi cause this condition, and their grains differ in colour. The patient complains of aching pain in the affected area. Mycetoma occurs around the World in both tropical and temperate regions, and was first described in India, where, however, whole areas are free of infection. There is an association between the disease and conditions of semi-aridity. It is found particularly in Africa, but is not uncommon in Mexico and Central America. Cases have been reported from Italy and South Vietnam. There is a good case for not walking bare-footed in many countries. Homoeopathic therapy includes:

(1) *Silicea 6 6h*
(2) Collect a small quantity of coloured granules from the discharging pus, and place in a small glass tube containing 90% alcohol (ethanol). Send to the homoeopathic pharmacist, requesting a *nosode* to be made from this material,

of potency *30c* (in the form of pilules or drops). Upon receipt, give the patient one dose of this preparation once daily in conjunction with prescription (1), given above.

Dermatitis verrucosa (Mossy foot/ Chromoblastomycosis)

This is caused by inoculation of a black mould into a wound, usually on the foot. It is mainly seen in South America in people working in bare feet. Thorns again are implicated, as with madura foot (see above). A small warty lesion is produced, which slowly enlarges. A fully established case (after several years) has many cauliflower-like masses attached to the skin, which bleed easily, and have a foul odour. There is little pain, but considerable irritation. Homoeopathic therapy includes:

(1) *Thuja 6 12h*
(2) Application of the following cream *12h*:
   Unguenti Emulsificantis Aquosi   *30g*
   Olei Melalucae Alternifoliorum   *15gtt*
   Thujae ø   *10gtt*

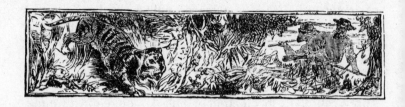

Section 18

COMMON INJURIES, EMERGENCIES AND INFECTIONS

Everyone, including children over 10 years of age, especially if travelling to far off places, should be encouraged to take a basic first-aid course. See also *Section 8* (thrush, cystitis), *Section 17* (sprains of ankle and knee, pulled muscle, muscular fatigue), and *Section 19* (eye injuries).

SOME COMMON INJURIES AND EMERGENCIES

Bruise (Contusion)
For bruises in general, take internally:

    Arnica 30 2h

Abrasions, Cuts, Wounds
The main risks are excessive bleeding and infection, including tetanus. All wounds, with the exception of superficial abrasions, should ideally be seen by a medical or paramedical practitioner. For the treatment of wounds inflicted by

animals, see *Section 15*. Otherwise, first-aid treatment is as follows:

(1) Flush with large amounts of soap and water, alcohol (eg vodka), or antiseptic solution (eg *Rose Water [triple]*).

(2) Arrest bleeding by pressure, and the internal use of the following remedy:

Arnica 30 ½h

(3) For the homoeopathic treatment of *psychological or physical shock*, see below under the appropriate headings.

(4) Apply either of the following on a clean dressing, to promote healing, renewing several times daily:

(a) *Cremor Calendulae 5%*
(b) *Calendula ø 1 part + clean water 9 parts*

(5) Additionally, for all wounds, except superficial abrasions, where the tetanus immunization status is inadequate or unknown, give the following internal remedy until a physician can be consulted [continue for 4 months in the absence of proper medical advice]:

Ledum 30 12h

(6) In certain situations there may be no clean water or antiseptic available with which to clean a wound. In arid areas of the Americas, the juice of the *cardon cactus (Pachycerius pectin-aboriginum)* may be used to the same end. Moreover, a piece of the flesh of this cactus applied to the wound, and held in place with a clean bandage, will arrest bleeding, rather like *Arnica*.

Burns

The best emergency treatment is the liberal application of the oily contents of a natural *vitamin E (d-Alpha Tocopheryl Acetate)* capsule. It should be applied as soon as possible, and reapplied every hour or two. It significantly reduces damage to the skin, and promotes healing. Alternatively, creams containing natural vitamin E are satisfactory, and may be applied with similar frequency (use either of the formulae given in *Section 12*).

Fracture

Usually evident by severe pain, considerable swelling, deformity, and loss of function (see also below under *sprained wrist*). Treat as follows:

(1) Immobilize fracture area, in order to prevent further damage. Use temporary wooden splints, if necessary.

(2) If patient is *psychologically or physically shocked*, treat as given below under those headings.

(3) Give the following, to control internal bleeding:

> *Arnica 30 ½h*

(4) Transport for medical attention.

(5) *After* reduction (realignment) of the fracture, give the following in order to promote union, and continue until this has occurred:

> *Symphytum 6 6h*

(6) The same prescription as given in (5) is excellent in cases of *non-union*.

Botanic casts for fractures

Virtually any plant that yields a non-irritant and hard-setting syrup can be used to form a cast. In Mexico, 'solda con solda', a tree-climbing arum lily, and 'tepeguaje', a tree of the bean family, are used for this purpose. Once the fracture is correctly aligned, the limb is wrapped in soft cloth followed by a layer of cotton or wild kapok. 1kg of tepeguaje bark is boiled in 5 litres of water, until 2 litres remain. The resultant liquid is strained, and then further boiled until a thick syrup is formed. Strips of material (gauze, sheeting, flannel) are saturated with the syrup, and are applied as one would a normal cast. As with all casts, it must be changed if the patient's fingers or toes become cold, white, blue, or numb.

Psychological shock

This results from either physical or mental trauma. The patient is conscious, but will exhibit any or all of the following: agitation, apprehension, disorientation, terror, nausea, sweating, pallor, rapid pulse, feeling faint. Irrespective of the cause, treat with either of the following, given *every 10 minutes*:

(1) *Aconite 30*

(2) *Bach Rescue Remedy*

[alternatively, in the case of physical trauma, use *Arnica 30* similarly]

Should the patient then *faint*, treat as for *physical shock* (see below).

Physical shock (Collapse)

The causes of this are numerous: simple faint, loss of blood, heart attack, snake bite, and so on. Obviously, expert medical assistance is desirable, but emergency treatment is within the capabilities of the ordinary citizen. The patient is either *semi-conscious* or *unconscious*, and the pulse feeble. The following measures must be carried out *immediately*, whatever the cause, even before the arrival of a physician:

(1) Place patient in *horizontal* position on one side. Lift up chin away from neck (tilt head back), to maintain airway.

(2) Ensure airway is clear. Remove vomit or food from mouth and nose, and remove any dentures.

(3) If the patient is *not breathing*, produce lung inflation by either *mouth-to-mouth* breathing (keeping patient's nostrils tightly closed with thumb and forefinger), or *mouth-to-nose* breathing (closing patient's mouth). This is best carried out with the patient in the supine position (on the back), with the head pulled backwards. The inflation rate should be approximately *12 times per minute*, allowing about 2 seconds for inflation, and about 3 seconds for spontaneous expiration (which occurs by elastic recoil of the chest wall). Should the action of the heart be feeble or undetectable, then external cardiac massage is required, but this is best left to those who have been trained properly in its use (hence, the value of first-aid courses).

(4) If the patient is *semiconscious*, give homoeopathic remedies as suggested for *psychological shock* (see above), but give them in liquid or powdered form. If, however, the patient is *unconscious*, give either of the following two remedies *every 10 minutes*:

(a) *Carbo vegetabilis 30* [crushed/liquid form]
(b) *Bach Rescue Remedy*

217

[note that (b) is generally useful for all types of shock, but (a) is a more powerful agent in serious cases of physical shock; with some exaggeration, it has been termed 'the homoeopathic corpse reviver']

Drowning
Proceed as for *physical shock* (see above).

Concussion
All patients receiving blows to the head should be seen by a physician. The following should be given as a matter of routine (even by physicians), until symptoms disappear:

Natrum sulphuricum 30 6h

Accidental overdose
It should go without saying that *all* medicines should be kept away from children. However, should accidental overdose or poisoning be suspected, bear in mind the following facts:

(1) All homoeopathic remedies bearing a potency number of 6c (6/6 CH), 12x (D12), or greater are *non-toxic*, even if taken in large quantities by small children. Artificially induced vomiting, and stomach wash-outs are *not* indicated! Merely reprehend the child. Similarly, Bach flower remedies in their diluted form, ready for use, are very safe.

(2) However, certain vitamins (notably *A, B6, D, E*), certain minerals (notably *iron*), certain homoeopathic mother tinctures (such as *Thuja* ø), and many orthodox drugs are potentially toxic if reasonable amounts are ingested. If accidental overdose is suspected, it is wise to induce vomiting artificially, by placing a finger down the throat, with the patient vertical, and head forward, in order to avoid the inhalation of vomit. In all cases, a physician should be consulted.

Sprained wrist
This may be treated along similar lines to those quoted for sprained ankle and twisted knee (see *Section 17*), with *Arnica 30* as the main homoeopathic remedy, or, in substitution, *Ruta graveolens 30*. It is important, however, not to

miss a fracture of the *scaphoid* bone, situated at the base of the thumb, for which plastering will be required fairly urgently. Ask the patient to actively extend his thumb. Two almost parallel tendons will appear at the base of the thumb where it joins the wrist, in line with the thumb nail. The depression between them is termed 'the anatomical snuff box'. Place your index finger in the 'snuff box', and press firmly. If any distinct pain or tenderness is felt by the patient, a fracture of the scaphoid is to be suspected, and this must be confirmed by X-ray. If you are in circumstances where medical help is unavailable, splint the wrist as best you can, and give *Symphytum 6*, as described above for *fractures* in general.

Tennis elbow and golfer's elbow
With tennis elbow, tenderness is experienced on the outer aspect of the elbow joint, accompanied by pain on move-ment. With golfer's elbow, the tenderness is on the inner aspect of the elbow joint. Contrary to popular opinion, neither of these conditions is to be regarded as a primary disorder of the elbow. Usually, their origin lies in minor dislocation of the vertebrae of the thoracic spine (that part of the backbone behind the chest). Pressure on the spinal nerves induces a referred pain to the elbow, and reactive muscle spasm occurs in this area. The muscle in spasm con-stricts its own blood supply, and inflammation results. What-ever therapy is given to the elbow, it will often fail, unless the displaced vertebrae are reduced by chiropractic or similar manipulation. As a complement to the latter, or until such can be procured, consider:

(1) *Rhus toxicodendron 30 6h*
(2) *Agaricus muscarius 6 6h*

Traumatic coccyalgia (Bruised tailbone)
Falls on the rump are not uncommon amongst skiers and ice sportsmen. Often the coccyx (tailbone) is intact, but occasionally may suffer a fairly unimportant fracture. In all cases, to reduce discomfort:

Hypericum 30 ½-4h

Crushed fingers
From car doors, or ball games:

> *Hypericum 30 ¼-4h*

General exhaustion
From exercise:

> *Arnica 30 ½h*

> [see also *heat exhaustion*, in *Section 12*]

Cutaneous foreign bodies (Splinters)
Splinters, thorns, or sea urchin spines (see *Section 15*) left in the skin are not only painful, but may also give rise to infection. The following assists in the expulsion of such foreign bodies, where surgical removal cannot be performed:

> *Silicea 6 6h*

> [it may be necessary to take this for many weeks]

Nosebleed (Epistaxis)
Whereas this may occur from a blow to the nose, it more commonly occurs spontaneously. In adults (especially the elderly), it may be a symptom of high blood pressure (hypertension). Emergency treatment is as follows:

(1) The patient should be seated in the upright position, with the head tilted forward, the soft part of the nose pinched firmly with finger and thumb, and the mouth open. Any blood that accumulates in the mouth should be spat out, and not swallowed.

(2) The patient should be reassured and calmed.

(3) The following remedy should be given (coarse granules, pilules, or tablets may be crunched between the teeth):

> *Ferrum phosphoricum 30 ¼h*

(4) Should the patient be excessively agitated, a dose of either of the following may be given between doses of the above remedy, as required:
(a) *Aconite 30*
(b) *Bach Rescue Remedy*

SOME COMMON INFECTIONS AND DISORDERS OF CHILDREN

Common cold and influenza
The following may be considered, either to abort the illness or hasten its end:

(1) Where the illness has been brought on by chilling, this remedy may be used at the onset (but is of little use once the illness is fully developed):

> *Aconite 30 1h*

(2) Alternatively, in general:

> *Zingiber ø 10–20 drops 4h*

> [reduce the dose for children]

(3) Alternatively, and in general, the following mixed remedy may be used *4h*:

> *Oscillococcinum 200*
> *Gelsemium 30*
> *Lemna minor 6*
> *Sepia 6*

(4) In addition to any of the above measures, either or both of the following nutritional supplements may be taken (adult doses quoted):
>   (a) *Zinc 15mg 12h* [reduce the dose if cramps occur]
>   (b) *Vitamin C 1000mg 4–6h*

Warning!: Certain serious illnesses may present with influenza-like symptoms, for which the treatment is quite different, and the services of a physician should be sought. Most importantly, any person returning from an endemic malaria zone with a fever or flu-like symptoms, should have a blood test carried out to eliminate the possibility of *malaria*. This matter should not be delayed. Typhoid, amongst others, may present similarly.

Acute bronchitis (Rattling chest)
Give the following mixture of remedies *6h*:

> *Antimonium tartaricum 6*

221

Oscillococcinum 200

Acute sinusitis (Blocked sinuses)

Thick catarrh, accompanied by pain and tenderness in the cheeks, or above the eyes:

(1) *Kali iodatum 30 6h*
(2) *Silicea 30 6h*

Acute tonsillitis (Severe sore throat)

The tonsils are red, sometimes with white spots. Consider the following:

(1) In general:

Mercurius corrosivus 6 6h

(2) Where the lymph glands of the upper neck are greatly enlarged and tender:

Phytolacca 30 6h

(3) Where, additionally, there is tenderness of the glands in the arm-pits and groins (glandular fever, or similar viral infection), the above prescriptions will often fail. Consider instead:

Glandular fever nosode 30 12h

(4) Where a *quinsy* (peritonsillar abscess) develops, as witnessed by gross enlargement of the tonsillar area, and severe pain, consider:
(a) *Lachesis 30 4h*
(b) *Silicea 30 4h*

Note: *Lassa fever* may present as a severe 'tonsillitis'. See *Section 24*, with regard to diagnosis and treatment.

Acute laryngitis (Loss of voice)

May be due to viral infections or misuse of the vocal cords:

Arum triphyllum 30 6h

Earache (Otalgia)

Perhaps the commonest cause of severe earache in children, without swelling or discharge, is *acute otitis media* (acute middle ear infection). If the condition is allowed to progress, the ear-drum will often rupture, with the appearance of pus in the outer ear, and a considerable reduction of pain. Treatment may include:

(1) Given early enough, a single dose of the following remedy will often abort an attack:

Medorrhinum 200

[another dose of the same may be repeated 12 hours later, but no more should be given after that]

(2) In the absence of the above remedy, and also of use in common fevers and *teething* in children, the following mixed remedy ('homoeopathic Calpol') may be given *½-2h*:

ABC 30

[*Aconite 30 + Belladonna 30 + Chamomilla 30*]

(see also *Section 16* [ear boils, otomycosis], and *mumps*, below)

Swimming pool earache (Chlorine otalgia)
Particularly in children, irritation of the eustachian tube, which leads from the middle ear to the throat, may cause repeated episodes of ear pain, possibly associated with secondary bacterial infection of the middle ear. This may be prevented as described for *chlorine conjunctivitis* (see *Section 19*). The attacks themselves are treated as given above under *earache (otalgia)*.

Toothache (Odontalgia)
Severe toothache warrants investigation by a dental surgeon. Frequently the problem is caused by either a dying pulp (nerve), or a dead pulp with abscess formation and swelling. Emergency treatment is as follows:

(1) *Hepar sulphuris 6 6h*
(2) If the tooth is sensitive to either heat or cold, and a cavity is present, insert a pledget of cotton-wool soaked in *Oleum Carophylli* (oil of cloves).

223

Infantile colic (Colicky babies)

Assuming no serious pathology, which is usually the case, try:

Colocynthis 30 6h

Mumps (Epidemic parotitis)

Painful swelling of salivary glands due to a virus. One or both parotid glands are usually involved, leading to swelling in front of and below the ear. In males, either or both testicles may become enlarged and painful. Incubation period: 14–21 days. Infectivity to others: from 1 day before symptoms appear, and up to 7 further days. Homoeopathic treatment:

(1) *Jaborandi 30 4h*
(2) Especially where testicular inflammation occurs:

Pulsatilla 6 4h

Measles (Rubeola)

A common viral infection of childhood, causing 1 million deaths world-wide each year (death rate 10% in developing countries). The child becomes unwell. About 2 days before the main rash occurs, *Koplik's spots appear in the mouth*, lasting 1–4 days. These resemble table salt crystals (on a red base), and are found on the inner surfaces of the cheeks. They are absolutely diagnostic of measles, and no other illness. The main rash, which is brick-red and blotchy, first appears on the face, and then includes the trunk. Incubation period: 10–14 days. Infectivity to others: from about 4 days before the onset of the main rash, lasting for the duration of the rash. The patient should be kept in darkened quarters. The following remedy will be found helpful in many cases, to reduce the severity of the disease, and to reduce the likelihood of serious complications:

Pulsatilla 6 4h

German Measles (Rubella)

A much lesser illness in children than measles (see above). The child is usually only mildly unwell. A pink rash appears suddenly, fading within 3 days. The lymph glands behind the ears and at the base of the skull become characteristically tender 5–10 days before the onset of the rash. Incubation period: 14–21 days. Infectivity to others: from 7 days before the rash to when the rash disappears. In adults, the disease may be more severe, with joint pains occurring. Women in early pregnancy, whose rubella immune status is inadequate, should avoid contact with possible cases. In general, the illness is so mild, it barely warrants any treatment. However, homoeopathically it may be treated as for *measles* (see above).

Chickenpox (Varicella)

The small pus-filled blisters of this viral disease are well-known to most parents. The rash is symmetrical, and is concentrated on the face, scalp, and trunk. Ulcerated lesions also occur in the throat. The blisters dry to produce crusts, which usually fall off within 7–14 days. Incubation period: 10–20 days. Infectivity to others: until all the crusts are detached. Chickenpox may be treated with the following two remedies, given *in alternation (alternately), every 2 hours*:

(1) *Rhus toxicodendron 30*
(2) *Antimonium tartaricum 6*

Shingles (Herpes zoster)

This disease, due to reactivation of a chickenpox virus, is not uncommon in adults, especially the elderly. The rash itself resembles chickenpox, with small blisters which become pus-filled, on a red base. However, unlike chickenpox, it usually is to be found only on one side of the body. The common sites are: the face, the abdomen, the rib-cage. It is accompanied by severe pain and irritation. The pain often precedes the rash by several days. The whole illness, without treatment, may take several weeks to resolve. Infectivity to others: as for chickenpox (see above). Homoeopathic treatment can do much to shorten this unpleasant illness, and reduce its severity:

(1) The main internal remedy:

225

Rhus toxicodendron 30 6h

(2) Where the rash is around the rib-cage, the following may be substituted:

Ranunculus bulbosus 30 6h

Rickettsialpox (Kew Gardens spotted fever)

A relatively rare disease, which may be confused with chickenpox. It is caused by a rickettsial organism harboured by mice, and is transmitted to man via infected mites. It has been described in the eastern USA, French Equatorial Africa, and the former USSR. Early lesions resemble chickenpox, but the throat is seldom ulcerated. The illness is mild, and often resolves in 10 days or so. Homoeopathic treatment might be considered along the lines given for chickenpox (see above).

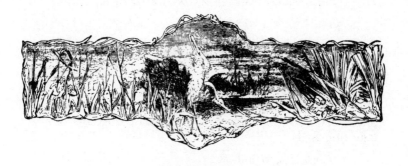

Section 19

EYE PROBLEMS

Always protect your eyes from the damaging effects of intense sunlight. Even seated under a beach parasol, there will be a great amount of ultraviolet radiation reflected from the sand, and white objects. With depletion of the ozone layer, these problems are exaggerated, and both cataract (opacity of the lens of the eye) and pterygium (see below) are becoming more common. Use both dark glasses and a peaked or brimmed hat to protect yourself. If you do wear corrective glasses, and you are venturing to remote places, always remember to take at least one spare pair with you.

Black eye
For blows to the eye from blunt objects, such as balls or fists:

(1) The best remedy for the pain:

Symphytum 30 1h

(2) Should the above fail to relieve the pain:

Hypericum 30 1h

(3) Thereafter, residual bruising may be dispelled by either of the following:

(a) *Ledum 30 4h*
(b) *Arnica 30 4h*

Foreign bodies

Dust, sand, or small insects may cause considerable irritation. To assist in their expulsion, and reduce discomfort, take internally:

Coccus cacti 30 ¼h

Eye-strain

From prolonged driving, or reading in bad light, often accompanied by headache:

Ruta graveolens 6 2h

Acute conjunctivitis

This is inflammation of the membrane (conjunctiva) that covers the white of the eye and the inner surfaces of the eyelids. The eye becomes red, itchy, sore, and watery, and there may be the production of yellow pus. It is important to differentiate acute conjunctivitis from other, more serious, disorders, such as acute glaucoma (increased eye pressure), acute uveitis (inflammation of the iris and associated structures), and corneal ulceration, for which expert help will be required. Fortunately, this is usually a relatively easy matter. The vision in acute conjunctivitis is not disturbed (if there is any minor disturbance of vision, it can be cleared by blinking), and any pain is mild. Often, both eyes are affected. In the severe disorders mentioned, vision is generally blurred (it cannot be cleared by blinking), the pain moderate to intense, and usually only one eye is affected. In *retinal detachment*, which requires urgent surgical attention, one eye is involved, which is neither red nor painful, but again vision is disturbed (as though a curtain had descended over it). Acute conjunctivitis with much itching and watery discharge is normally of allergic origin, and is, most frequently, a manifestation of hay-fever. Fortunately, when those who suffer from the latter go abroad, the condition frequently fails to appear. This is because the pollens they experience are different from those at home. However, after a prolonged stay, they often succeed in becoming allergic to these as well. Acute conjunctivitis with *pus* is more likely of infective origin. It may be contracted via dirty towels, fingers, or contaminated foreign bodies. So-called *eye flies* may be responsible for *epidemic conjunctivitis* in India, Sri Lanka, Java and the southern USA. The treatment of acute conjunctivitis may proceed along the following lines:

(1) Use the following eye lotion, *1–2 drops each eye 4h* (it should be made up freshly every few days, and kept cool):

Rose Water (triple)	*5ml (1 teaspoon)*
Boiled water	*5ml (1 teaspoon)*
Euphrasia ∅	*2 drops*

(2) If the above is unavailable, use *cold tea* similarly.
(3) Additionally, internal remedies should be given:
    (a) Where the discharge is watery, or there is little pus, give the following combination of remedies *4h*:

        Euphrasia 30
        Allium cepa 30

    (b) Where there is profuse pus:

        Argentum nitricum 30 4h

    [see also *snow blindness, swimmer's eye, and trachoma*, below]

Snow blindness (Glare conjunctivitis)
This inflammatory condition is found in skiers and mountaineers (see *Section 13*). Treatment:

(1) Use *eye-drops*, as suggested above for *acute conjunctivitis*.
(2) Additionally, give internally either of the following:
    (a) *Aconite 30 4h*
    (b) *Cicuta virosa 30 4h*

Swimmer's eye (Chlorine conjunctivitis)
An acute conjunctivitis due to contact with chlorinated water used in swimming pools. Certain individuals are particularly prone to this problem, and are advised to wear swimming

goggles. However, the condition can largely be prevented by giving the following remedy in *3 doses: 1 dose one hour before swimming, 1 dose immediately before swimming, 1 dose on leaving the pool:*

Chlorum 8x(D8)

Sty[e] (Hordeolum)

This is a common staphylococcal infection of the eyelid. An acutely tender, swollen and red area appears on the margin of the upper or lower eyelid. It may be treated as follows:

(1) Initially:

Pulsatilla 6 4h

(2) Subsequently, after the pain and redness are much reduced:

Staphysagria 6 6h

Pterygium

A condition in which a triangular area of fleshy conjunctiva extends towards the cornea, with the apex towards the pupil. It is usually situated on the nasal side of the eye, and exposure to wind, dust, sand, and sun are contributory to its development. Irritation may be controlled by the use of eye drops (use the formulation given above under *acute conjunctivitis*). As it enlarges, so it encroaches upon the cornea, causing disturbance of vision. Folk treatment using powdered shells is useless and harmful. Surgical removal provides an immediate solution, but recurrences are common. Homoeopathic remedies may be tried as an alternative, or in conjunction with surgery, in the hope of preventing relapse:

(1) *Ratanhia 6 12h*
(2) Should the above fail after 4 weeks of treatment:

Zincum metallicum 6 12h

Tropical blindness

The major causes of blindness in the tropics are: *nutritional deficiency, trachoma,* and *onchocerciasis (river blindness).*

These are discussed below. Other important causes include: bacterial conjunctivitis (see above), leprosy, cataract (opacity of the lens), and atrophy (wasting) of the optic nerve.

Nutritional blindness

Various nutritional deficiency states are implicated in the occurrence of eye problems in developing countries. These deficiencies include those of vitamin B1, vitamin B2, vitamin B12, nicotinic acid, folic acid, vitamin C, and vitamin D. However, the most important is *vitamin A deficiency*, produced by an inadequate diet. This is most common in children of 2–10 years of age, and if not identified early enough and treated, permanent blindness may result. It is important, therefore, to recognise the signs of this disease:

(1) Initially, *night blindness*. Inability to see in the dark as well as others. In dim light, the child readily stumbles over objects.

(2) Later, *dry eyes (xerosis)*. The temporal (outer) side of the white of each eye becomes dull and wrinkled.

(3) Patches of grey bubbles, known as *Bitot's spots* may appear on the white of the eye (these spots in themselves do not specifically confirm the diagnosis of vitamin A deficiency, since they may be caused by a variety of other deficiency states).

(4) As the condition advances, so the cornea becomes dry, dull, and sometimes pitted.

(5) Later, the cornea softens, and may bulge or burst, usually without pain. Infection and scarring may occur. The blindness worsens.

(6) Xerosis often begins, or worsens during the course of another illness, such as measles, dysentery, and tuberculosis. It is important, therefore, to carefully examine the eyes of all ill and underweight children.

The condition is *prevented* by supplying adequate quantities of food rich in vitamin A, or supplements of the same:

(A) Breast feeding of babies is to be encouraged. This should be continued for up to 2 years, where possible.

231

(B) After the child has attained 6 months of age, introduce,
     according to availability:
     (a) **Dark green, leafy vegetables.**
     (b) **Yellow and red vegetables.**
     (c) Yellow and red fruits.
     (d) Eggs, liver, kidneys, whole milk.
(C) If these foods are unavailable, give one capsule of vita-
     min A 200,000IU (retinol 60mg) *once every 6 months*.
     This must not be given to children under 6 months of
     age.

The treatment of the established condition involves the
administration of vitamin A supplementation, either orally,
or by injection:

(1) Early cases of night blindness and xerosis. Treat as
given in (C) above. Sometimes 'de-worming' is helpful (see
ascariasis in *Section 27*).

(2) More severe cases, but without corneal changes,
should receive a single dose of vitamin A 200,000IU (retinol
60mg), which may be repeated *one week later* if there is no
improvement. **Excesses of vitamin A are toxic**. No more than
200,000IU (1 capsule of retinol 60mg) should be given per
week, and a total dose of 1,000,000IU (5 capsules of retinol
60mg) should not be exceeded.

(3) If the cornea is dull, pitted, or bulging, a single intra-
muscular *injection* of vitamin A 100,000IU (retinyl palmi-
tate) should be given, the eyes bandaged, and medical help
sought. If the injection is unavailable, give oral doses as
described immediately above.

Trachoma
This is a chronic infective (chlamydial) conjunctivitis, associated with poor nutrition and inadequate hygiene. Whilst it
is more common in the tropics, it occurs elsewhere, where
unsanitary conditions prevail. It is spread by touch, flies,
dust, and fine sand. Even in Australia it is found amongst
aborigines who live in unhygienic circumstances. It is responsible for more cases of blindness than any other disease.
Neither are travellers immune who care to live roughly. It
is found in the Balkans (especially Bulgaria), southern

Spain, the eastern Mediterranean (especially Jordan and Lebanon), Arabia, Iran, Morocco, Tunisia, Egypt, Sudan, India, China, Indonesia, the Pacific Archipelago, and Japan. It is common in most African countries, with the exception of Liberia and Zaire, where most of the population live in the rain forest, and the dust and fine sand that carry the infection through the air are not conspicuous.

The initial signs of trachoma are similar to those of *acute conjunctivitis* (see above). The eyes are red and watery. After a month or longer, pink-grey lumps, termed *follicles*, appear on the inside of the upper eyelids. The eyelids must be everted to see these. The white of the eye is mildly inflamed, and, upon close inspection, the top of the cornea appears grey. This latter phenomenon is due to invasion of the cornea by new blood vessels and infiltrate, termed *pannus*. The combination of *follicles plus pannus* is confirmatory of trachoma. After several years, the follicles tend to disappear, leaving white scars, which thicken and deform the eyelids. Where such deformity pulls the eyelashes on to the cornea, the latter is scratched, scarring occurs, and blindness follows.

Orthodox therapy includes antibiotic therapy (which is not without problems), and surgery to correct deformity. Homoeopathic treatment includes:

(1) At the onset, trachoma will appear very similar to watery *acute conjunctivitis*, and treatment may be given along the same lines as suggested for that condition (see above).

(2) With the development of follicles and pannus:
    (a) *Kali bichromicum 6 12h*
    (b) *Alumina 6 12h*

(3) In the later stages, with scarring of the eyelid:
    (a) *Graphites 6 12h*
    (b) *Borax 6 12h*

(4) Eye-drops of the same formulation as given for *acute conjunctivitis* (see above) may be useful at any stage.

Onchocerciasis (River blindness)

This disease is found in many parts of Africa, southern Mexico, Guatemala, Colombia, Venezuela, and northern

Brazil. The infective organism is a parasitic nematode worm transmitted by the bite of certain hump-backed flies, known as *black flies*. These flies breed in fast flowing water, and the clearance of vegetation from the banks of streams is helpful in reducing their numbers. These flies usually bite during the day, during which time it is safer not to sleep outdoors. *Several months* after an effective bite, painless lumps (no more than 3–6) appear on the body, which slowly grow to a size of 2–3cm (about 1in) in diameter. In Africa, the lumps are usually found on the lower body and thighs, whereas in the Americas, they are most common on the head and upper body. Severe itching may be caused by an allergic response to the worms, and areas of the skin become thickened, scaly, and dark. Eye disorders are a common sequel, but are less likely in transient visitors with light infection. Initially, there may be redness and watering. Inflammation of the iris, with pain and visual disturbance, follows. The cornea becomes dull, pitted, and scarred. The patient is rendered blind. Fortunately, many people in endemic areas live in balance with the parasite, and do not exhibit serious symptoms. Orthodox treatment includes the use of drugs to kill the worms, but there may be dangerous side effects. Homoeopathically, remedies may be given for the various individual eye problems, but, on a more general basis, the remedy *Kali iodatum 30 12h* may be of help in some cases, and *Sulphur 6 12h* in others.

African eye worm (Loiasis/Loa loa)

See Section 27

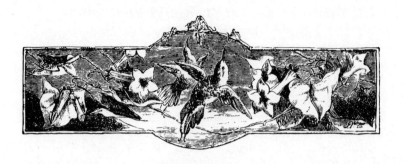

Section 20

MALARIA

Malaria, formerly known as *intermittent fever* or *The Ague*, is a parasitic disease generally transmitted via the bite of the female *Anopheles* mosquito, and occasionally by blood transfusion, or communal needle techniques. It may also be transmitted to the human foetus via the placenta. Most infections are acquired in the tropics and subtropics, where malaria is endemic; but it is not unknown for infection to occur from the bite of a 'rogue' mosquito within an aircraft which has refueled in, or has previously visited an endemic area. Malaria is responsible for over one million deaths world-wide each year, and the matter of its prevention is discussed in *Sections 3 and 14* of the manual.

Distribution of malaria

Whilst malaria is endemic in many countries, it should be understood that the risk to the traveller may vary according to the season and locality. Many urban areas are very safe in this respect, as are some areas of high altitude (malaria does not occur above 2500 metres/8200ft). Full information concerning these matters may be obtained by telephoning the Malaria Reference Laboratory of the UK (071-636 7921). If you are visiting any of the areas listed below you should obtain such advice (Ru = risk only in rural areas; Se = seasonal risk only):

Afghanistan [Se], Angola, Argentina [Ru], Bangladesh, Belize, Benin, Bhutan, Bolivia, Botswana [Se], Brazil [Ru], Burkino Faso, Burma, Burundi, Cambodia, Cameroon, Canal Zone (Panama), Central African Republic, Chad, China [Ru], Colombia, Congo, Costa Rica, Djibouti, Dominican Republic, Ecuador, Egypt [Se], El Salvador, Equatorial Guinea, Ethiopia, Gabon, Gambia, Ghana, Guatemala, Guiana (French), Guinea, Guinea Bissau, Guyana, Haiti, Honduras, India, Indonesia, Iran, Iraq [Ru], Ivory Coast, Kenya, Laos (Lao), Liberia, Libya [Se], Madagascar, Malawi, Malaysia [Ru], Mali, Mauritania, Mauritius [Ru], Mexico [Ru], Mozambique, Namibia, Nepal, Nicaragua, Niger, Nigeria, Oman, Pakistan, Panama, Papua New Guinea, Paraguay [Ru], Peru, Philippines, Rwanda, Sao Tomé and Principe, Saudi Arabia [Se], Senegal, Sierra Leone, Solomon Islands, Somalia, South Africa [Ru], Sri Lanka, Sudan, Surinam, Swaziland, Syria [Se], Tanzania, Thailand [Ru], Togo, Turkey [Ru/Se], Uganda, United Arab Emirates [Ru/Se], Vanuatu, Venezuela [Ru], Vietnam, Yemen (North), Yemen (South), Zaire, Zambia, Zimbabwe.

Presenting symptoms of malaria

Over 2000 cases of malaria are imported into the UK each year, with a progressive increase in mortality. The early recognition of malarial symptoms is of the utmost importance, not only for the resident of an endemic area, but also for the casual traveller, since swift treatment may be life-saving in the more pernicious varieties of this disease (see below). Even those who have taken the indicated orthodox prophylaxis may succumb, as has been mentioned in *Section 3*. The three most common presenting symptoms are:

> **Headache**
> **Fever**
> **Rigor (shivering fit/chill)**

Other common presenting symptoms include:

Diarrhoea
Vomiting
Cough
Malaise (feeling unwell)
Myalgia (muscle pains)
Jaundice (skin and whites of eyes go yellow)

It is quite possible to confuse malaria with influenza, gastro-enteritis, or hepatitis. The examination of a *blood film* for the presence of malarial parasites is of great importance in diagnostic differentiation.

Benign versus malignant malaria
Malaria is caused by four different types of protozoan parasite. *Plasmodium vivax, ovale and malariae* produce so-called *benign* malaria, characterised by recurrent fevers, continuing for months or years, even after the patient has quit the malaria zone, and only occasionally causing death, usually by rupture of the spleen. More deadly, however, is *malignant* malaria produced by *Plasmodium falciparum*, which is often life-threatening, and a grave medical emergency.

Benign malaria
The usual incubation period is 12–40 days, but the onset may be delayed for over one year, especially in those who have been taking prophylactic drugs. Initial (prodromal) symptoms may include malaise, fever, lack of appetite, perversion of taste (aversion to coffee or tobacco), diarrhoea, vomiting, and myalgia (muscle pains); none of which is absolutely diagnostic of malaria. Subsequently, however, there is a change towards the manifestation of recurrent *characteristic* attacks (paroxysms), usually lasting for several to many hours, and which may be divided into three phases:

(1) *Cold phase.* The patient feels intensely cold, and shivers or shakes. This phase lasts from about 15 minutes to 1 hour.

(2) *Hot phase.* The patient feels intensely hot and weak. The face is flushed. There is fever, with a temperature of up to 41°C (105.8°F). There may be intense thirst, vomiting,

abdominal pain, an increased flow of urine, or delirium. This phase often lasts 4–6 hours.

(3) *Sweating phase*. Profuse sweating occurs for 1–2 hours, and the temperature returns to normal. The patient then feels weak, but generally not too unwell – until the next attack!

The frequency with which these attacks occur is dependent upon the species of parasite involved. Vivax and ovale malaria are extremely similar, and, after an initial period of irregular attacks, settle down to a periodicity of one every 48 hours. This is termed *benign tertian* malaria, since the attacks occur every third day. In contrast, malariae malaria (that caused by Plasmodium malariae), has a periodicity of 72 hours. This is termed *quartan* malaria, in that the attacks occur every fourth day.

As a result of these attacks, there may develop anaemia, mild jaundice, and enlargement of the liver and spleen, which latter, as has been mentioned above, may rupture, with fatal consequences. Occasionally, a severe kidney disorder may arise (malaria nephrosis). Frequent attacks of herpes simplex (cold sores) are not uncommon.

Even without treatment, the patient usually enters a phase of remission, where fever is absent, which lasts approximately 2–3 months. Following this, and for a period of 8–50 years, relapses often occur and recur with similar frequency, in the absence of satisfactory therapy. Repatriation to a cooler climate may be helpful, but it is common for relapses to be precipitated by subsequent visits to hot countries.

Malignant malaria (Falciparum malaria)
Regrettably, this disease is on the increase. Whilst the falciparum parasite is to be found throughout the malaria zones of the World, the greatest risk is to those who visit West Africa. The usual incubation period for this form of malaria is 9–14 days. Certainly 95% of those infected develop symptoms within one month. More rarely, symptoms may be delayed for up to one year, delay again being more likely in those on prophylactic drugs. The fever is often irregular,

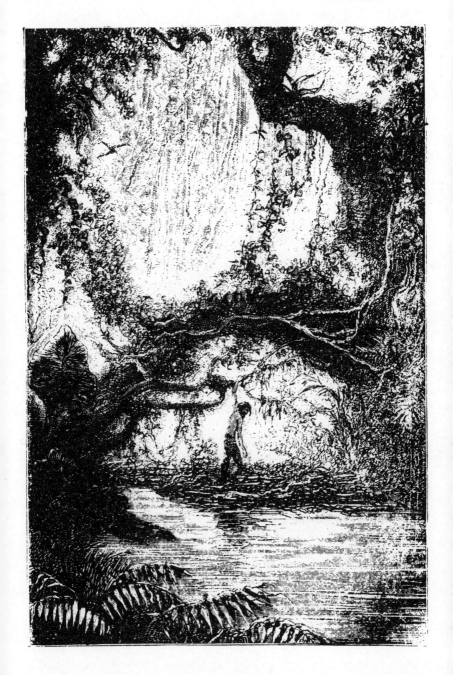

239

and usually lacks the characteristic periodicity one associates with established benign malaria (see above). If any periodicity develops, it may be of the *subtertian* type – slightly more often than every third day. The term *malignant tertian* is sometimes applied to this disease, to differentiate it from the *benign tertian* type described above. The temperature may be persistently elevated, or, less commonly, it may be normal. Nausea, vomiting, myalgia (muscle pains), headache, loose cough, and confusion may occur. Diarrhoea is uncommon, and shaking or shivering are often absent. In severe cases, which are by no means uncommon, profound jaundice (mild in benign malaria), profound anaemia, hypoglycaemia (low blood sugar), pulmonary oedema (pulmonary edema/fluid on the lungs), and physical shock (circulatory collapse/*algid malaria*) may occur. Cerebral malaria is a particularly dire effect, characterised by unrousable coma, often accompanied by epileptiform fits. Strangely, if recovery from cerebral malaria does occur, there is seldom any residual neurological deficit. Enlargement of the spleen may occur, but is an inconstant phenomenon. *Blackwater fever* is now a rare complication of malignant malaria, and is characterised by the passage of extremely dark urine, resulting from the release of haemoglobin (oxygen-carrying pigment) from the red blood cells broken down by the parasite. It is now believed that this disorder is seldom associated with mortality.

Without satisfactory treatment, an initial attack of malignant malaria often results in death from one complication or another. If the patient survives, there is a residual anaemia, and some degree of immunity to the disease. Repeated attacks may, however, recur over the following twelve months, which, in the absence of reinfection, spontaneously disappear. The immunity conferred by an initial infection with falciparum parasites is, unfortunately, short-lived, and repeated infection is *desirable* in order to confer a continuing high level of protection.

Mixed malarial infections
Double infections with *Plasmodium vivax and falciparum*, or with *Plasmodium vivax and malariae* are not uncommon

in certain areas (eg India, Burma, Sri Lanka). These may give rise to complex symptomatic pictures. *Quotidian* malaria, characterised by the *daily* recurrence of fever, may be produced by such mixed infection.

Babesiosis (Piroplasmosis)

Babesia are protozoan organisms that infect cattle, dogs, other animals, and man. They may produce an illness resembling malaria, which is mild and not fatal, or a more severe illness resembling blackwater fever (see above), with fever and jaundice. Cases have been reported from the former Yugoslavia, Eire, the USA, and Scotland. A tick vector has been identified in the milder cases (USA). Homoeopathic treatment might be effected upon the lines given below for malaria.

Homoeopathic treatment of malarial attacks

I must preface my comments by stating that all likely cases of malaria should be referred to an experienced physician, where possible; this matter being all the more important in those of suspected malignant malaria. Since the malarial parasites are becoming increasingly and alarmingly more resistant to the action of orthodox drugs, it follows that my homoeopathic remarks are directed not only to those for whom homoeopathic treatment is the only possibility, but also to the enlightened physician.

Treatment of the malarial attack should begin as early as possible, even in the absence of a confirmatory blood test. It may even be started in the phase of prodromal symptoms, before the onset of more frank symptoms of malaria. If you suspect malaria as a possibility, do not await the development of the characteristic periodicity of the disorder before beginning treatment (such periodicity is often absent in cases of malignant malaria). With the exception of cases with serious complications, such as algid or cerebral malaria, the following treatment plan may be instituted:

(1) Three homoeopathic remedies are particularly important with regard to treatment. These are: *Arsenicum album*, *Pulsatilla*, and *Nux vomica*. Commence treatment with a triple alternation of these remedies, eg:
    10.30am: *Arsenicum album 6*
    11.00am: *Pulsatilla 6*

241

11.30am: *Nux vomica 6*
12 noon: *Arsenicum album 6, etc.*

Notes:

(a) If treatment is started in a cold phase of an attack (when there is shivering), the sequence should begin with *Nux vomica*: *Nux vom, Ars alb, Puls, Nux vom, etc.*

(b) If treatment is started at any phase other than a cold one, the sequence should begin with *Arsenicum album*: *Ars alb, Puls, Nux vom, Ars alb, etc.*

(c) The frequency of alternation of the remedies, or interval between doses, may be from *½ hour to 2 hours*, depending upon the severity of the case, and response. If in doubt, institute ½-hourly alternation.

(d) Should any or all of the remedies be unavailable in a 6th potency, higher potencies (eg 30) may be employed in the alternation. Even so, the interval between doses should be as specified above.

(e) Treatment by this method, provided serious complications do not develop (eg algid or cerebral malaria), should be continued until the end of the attack.

(f) The prescription may be deemed successful if any of the following changes occur: reduction in severity of the treated attack (compared with previous attacks), prolongation of the interval between the treated attack and any subsequent attack, reduction in severity of the subsequent attack.

(g) If deemed successful, the same alternation may be employed to treat any subsequent attacks.

(2) Should the method described in (1) be unsuccessful, then other remedies should be considered. In the case of the malarial attack without serious complications, one or two remedies should be selected from the following list, depending upon the individualized symptoms of the case (some leading indications for each remedy are stated):

(a) *Eupatorium perfoliatum 6.* Severe bone pains. Nausea and vomiting as the cold (shivering) phase passes. Feeling of pressure over the skull, or heaviness over the forehead. In many cases sensitive to this remedy, a sweating phase is virtually absent.

(b) *Gelsemium 6*. Marked flush of the face during the hot phase. Absence of thirst (or normal thirst) in all phases. Bruised feeling of the muscles. The chill (shivering) runs up the back.

(c) *Rhus toxicodendron 6*. Urticaria (nettle-rash/ hives) with violent itching and restlessness during the hot (raised temperature) phase, passing off in the sweating phase. Yellow, watery stool in the hot phase. Severe pains in the joints.

(d) *Apis mellifica 6*. Cold (shivering) phase ushered by sudden and violent vomiting. Urticaria (nettle-rash/hives) spreads over head and trunk as the cold (shivering) phase subsides, accompanied by swelling of lips and face. Pains in the joints (may be severe).

(e) *Chininum sulphuricum 6*. Ringing in the ears during the cold (shivering) phase. Great tenderness of spine, aggravated by touch or pressure. Marked periodicity of attacks.

(f) *Ipecacuanha 6*. Marked nausea. Tongue thickly coated with yellowish fur. Excessive salivation.

The presence of at least two characteristic symptoms is required to identify the probable remedy. If one of the above remedies is clearly indicated, it may be initially given *2h*. If two seem equally indicated, they should be given in alternation, with a initial dosage interval of *1 hour*. Again, alternative potencies may be used to that suggested above, without altering the timing of the dose repetition.

(3) In cases without serious complications, such as algid or cerebral malaria, which are, however, unresponsive to (1) and (2), a single dose of *Natrum muriaticum 200* should be given to 'clear' the case – that is to say, to change the symptomatic picture to one where either methods (1) or (2) might become applicable. This remedy should be administered immediately after the conclusion of an attack. The technique is particularly useful in cases that have become symptomatically distorted by the administration of partially effective orthodox drugs. Once the symptomatic picture has been 'cleared', method (1) should be reapplied to the case, followed by (2), should it fail.

(4) Cases which present with or develop serious complications will require expert medical attention, where available.

Cerebral malaria
The following homoeopathic remedies may be considered: Stramonium, Hyoscyamus, Belladonna, Opium.

Algid malaria
The following homoeopathic remedies may be considered: Veratrum album, Carbo vegetabilis, Camphora, Arsenicum album. Frequent repetition (every 10–15 minutes) is indicated.

Homoeopathic treatment in remission
Once the initial attacks of malaria have been subdued, the patient enters a phase of apparent remission. In this stage it is advisable to give other homoeopathic remedies in order to prevent or modify relapse, to reduce the likelihood of major reinfection, and to treat any enlargement of the spleen:

(1) In general, give *both*:
  (a) *Cinchona officinalis 30 12h*
  (b) *Malaria officinalis 30, one dose morning and evening [about 12 hours apart] on a particular day each week [eg Saturday] – on this day do not take the Cinchona officinalis.*

  [this prescription may be continued for many weeks or months]

(2) In some cases, the spleen will be enlarged, and this is detectable on abdominal examination by the physician. Even without examination, it may be suspected if there is discomfort in the upper abdomen under the *left* side of the rib-cage. In these circumstances, either of the following remedies should be prescribed, in addition to those given above in (1), for many months:
  (a) *Ceanothus americanus 6 12h*
  (b) *Quercus glandium spiritus ø 10 drops 6h*

  [reduce the dose of (b) for children]

(3) Having once suffered from attacks of malaria, and

having been repatriated to cooler climates, certain individuals will only exhibit relapse when visiting the tropics or subtropics. This phenomenon is not due to reinfection, but due to reactivation of the dormant disease. It may be prevented by giving:

Cinchona officinalis 30 12h

[from 2 weeks before the trip to 6 weeks after return; this prescription may be taken in preference to the *8x* suggested in *Section 3*, and usefully combined with *Malaria officinalis*, as stated in that section of the manual]

Katayama fever

This is yet another disorder that may be diagnostically confused with malaria. It occurs in association with bilharziasis, and is discussed in the section of the manual that immediately follows. It is readily differentiated from malaria by a simple blood test.

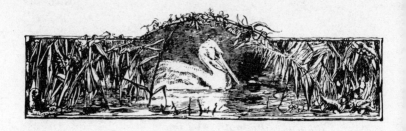

BILHARZIASIS
(SCHISTOSOMIASIS)

In that over 200 million people suffer this infection, and in view of its risk to travellers, it warrants our special attention. *Schistosomes* are blood flukes (flatworms), in maturity approximately 1–2cm (less than 1in) long, which inhabit the veins of the intestine or bladder of the human host. Here they lay their numerous eggs, which cause great irritation to the tissues, and pass via the *faeces* or *urine* to the outside world. Upon contact with fresh water, larval forms (miricidia) emerge from the eggs which then infect certain species of aquatic snail. Within the latter they develop into *cercariae*, immature forms only barely visible to the naked juvenile eye, which quit the snail in order to seek out and infect the human organism. Swimming freely through fresh water, and contacting a suitable host, they burrow through the skin, from where they migrate to grow to maturity.

Perversely, the growth of irrigation schemes to improve the agricultural competence, and thus nutrition, of the inhabitants of developing countries has significantly increased the prevalence of this serious disorder.

Avoidance

All travellers to endemic bilharziasis areas (see below) are at risk if they contact the water of lakes, streams, rivers, or ponds. Placing a single hand in such water may be disastrous. Particularly vulnerable are those who expose a large area of the skin to contaminated water, such as swimmers, water-skiers, canoeists, and wind-surfers. Since baboons harbour one variety of schistosome (*Schistosoma mansoni*) which also affects man, even water far removed from human habitation may be hazardous. Heavily polluted water, though dangerous in other respects, is usually free of cercariae. Human schistosomes are not to be found in salt or brackish water, but non-human varieties causing severe 'swimmer's itch' may be present (see *Section 16*). The use of wet-suits and rubber boots offers some measure of protection. Wearing long trousers and long-sleeved shirts provides a sensible barrier for those crossing streams or going on boats. Cercariae cannot survive in the absence of water; hence, rapid drying of skin, wet-suit, boots, or clothing is advisable, and this should be carried out at the earliest possible opportunity. Neglected swimming pools are a hazard, since they may contain aquatic snails. Water which has been chlorinated, or that which is snail-free and stored for 48 hours is safe. When crossing streams or rivers near human habitation, cross upstream of the latter rather than downstream. Water immediately behind a dam is often heavily contaminated with snails and cercariae.

Types and distribution of bilharziasis

The type of disease produced, and its geographical distribution varies according to the species of schistosome.

Schistosoma haematobium causes urinary schistosomiasis, also known as *bilharzia*. There is involvement of the bladder and related organs. It is found in many parts of Africa (including South Africa), Madagascar, Mauritius, the near East, and parts of Arabia. The River Nile is particularly hazardous. Mixed infections of *S. haematobium* and *S. mansoni* may occur.

In contrast, *Schistosoma mansoni* and *Schistosoma japonicum* cause disease of the bowel and the liver. *S. mansoni* is mainly endemic in Africa and Madagascar, but is also to be found in northeastern South America (especially Brazil), the Caribbean, and Arabia. *S. japonicum* is found in China, the Philippines, Sulawesi, and Japan.

Schistosoma intercalatum, which is found in Central and West Africa and Sao Tomé in the Gulf of Guinea, produces a disease similar to, but milder than that produced by *S. mansoni*. *Schistosoma mekongi*, found along the lower Mekong River, is similar to *S. japonicum* in its disease potential.

Effects of cercarial penetration

Soon after penetration of the skin by the immature schistosome, there may develop a sensation of tingling, followed by the development of an itchy rash (swimmer's/fisherman's itch). The rash produced by human schistosomes (with the exception of *Schistosoma japonicum*) is relatively insignificant compared with that produced by non-human varieties, which do not migrate into deeper tissues, and die under the skin (see *Section 16*). In many instances this reaction either goes unnoticed, or is frankly absent. Travellers to endemic areas are more likely to experience 'the itch' than those who are resident.

Disease caused by S. haematobium

After cercarial penetration of the skin, there is an incubation period of approximately 2–24 months. The illness often then begins with a mild fever, general weakness, and extreme exhaustion. With or without these initial symptoms, the *characteristic* index of the disorder appears – the **painless passage of blood in the urine**, especially at the end of urination. Pain is relatively uncommon, but may present as a dull ache above the pubic bone or burning at the tip of the penis. Frequency and urgency of urination may be experienced. The passage of blood in the stools can occur in some cases. Later complications include: cystitis, thickening of the bladder wall, kidney stones, inflammation of the pelvic organs (including the prostate and internal female genital structures), polyp formation (growths with stalks), cancer of the bladder, and heart failure. Serious complications are more likely in those subject to repeated invasion by schisto-somes. The diagnosis of urinary bilharziasis is readily con-firmed by finding the characteristic fluke eggs in the urine.

Disease caused by S. mansoni

This infection carries a significantly higher mortality than that described above. Significant symptoms develop 3–8 weeks after cercarial penetration. There is a sudden onset of malaise (feeling unwell), fever, cough, diarrhoea, and urticaria (nettle-rash/hives). This is termed *Katayama fever (or syndrome)*, and is generally seen in those who have not been brought up in an endemic area. There may be some confusion with malaria (see *Section 20*) or typhoid (see *Section 23*), but a simple blood test will differentiate (malarial parasites are absent, and there is an increase in those white cells known as *eosinophils*). Katayama fever is generally mild in this infection, and disappears. Involvement of the bowel wall leads to the passage of blood and mucus, resem-bling ulcerative colitis or other forms of dysentery (see *Section 10*). Characteristic eggs will be found in stool specimens. The liver and spleen may become enlarged, anaemia may be present, and severe kidney disease (glomerular nephritis) or heart failure may ensue.

Disease caused by S. japonicum

In regions where the water is highly contaminated with cer-cariae, this disease is generally more severe than that caused by *S. mansoni*. The initial dermatitis and irritation caused by the penetration of the skin may be intense. Some weeks later there develops Katayama fever (see above) of great severity, with marked urticaria (nettle-rash/hives). Fatalities may occur. The passage of blood in the stools may be pro-longed, and enlargement of the liver and spleen may ensue. Some cases develop epilepsy or a drum-like distention of the abdomen as the first serious presenting symptom.

Conversely, in the Philippines and Indonesia, where in-fection is less intense, the whole disease is usually much milder.

African eosinophilia

The occurrence of a raised eosinophil count in an unwell person who either resides in Africa, or has recently visited that country, is highly suggestive of worm infection, including bilharziasis.

Homoeopathic preventative measures

Whereas there is no orthodox immunization technique for bilharziasis, there is available a preventative method provided by homoeopathy, and this must be recommended to all those who put themselves at risk, albeit unproven as yet (see *Section 3*). I shall, however, not repeat the errors of my conventional colleagues in placing total reliance on any particular medicine (or medicines), but insist that the various methods of avoidance listed in the initial part of this section should be followed, where possible, as an adjunct (see above). Where exposure to water contaminated with schistosomes is a distinct possibility, as determined by geography, the following should be taken:

Caeruleum methylenum 3x 7 drops 12h

With regard to this prescription, the following observations should be made:

(1) Where the exposure to contaminated water is predictable (such as a forthcoming canoe race, or expedition), the prescription should be taken for a period extending from 2 days before to 3 days after the event.

(2) Where what appears to be 'swimmer's itch' develops in an endemic bilharziasis area, or where there has been significant exposure to the waters of such an area (eg falling in the water behind a dam), even in the absence of 'swimmer's itch', the above prescription should be taken for at least 8 weeks following the event.

(3) The dose should be reduced for children: give *1 drop per 10kg (22lb) body weight 12h*.

(4) Avoid this prescription in the first 3 months of pregnancy.

(5) Those suffering from *G-6-PD deficiency* should not take this prescription (see *Sections 2 and 11*).

(6) Adhere to the stated potency of *3x*.

Homoeopathic treatment of bilharziasis
Medical assistance should be sought in all cases of suspected bilharziasis. Orthodox treatment is available, but has its limitations. Most homoeopathic experience has been gained in the treatment of *S. haematobium* infections, which cause complications in the urinary tract, prostate, and the female genital organs. The therapeutic observations that follow are directed towards those with both medical training and some knowledge of homoeopathy:

(1) Whilst individualisation of each case, where possible, renders the best results, and though the individual response to the infection can be, homoeopathically speaking, fairly diverse, nevertheless certain remedies have won their laurels in the treatment of bilharziasis.

(2) As a basis for treatment, virtually all cases should be given:

Caeruleum methylenum 3x 7 drops 6h

Exceptions and provisos are as stated above with regard to homoeopathic prevention. The dose for children would be *1 drop per 10kg (22lb) body weight 6h*. This remedy should be given for an extended period, and in conjunction with any other indicated remedies given below.

(3) The frequency of dose repetition of the remedies that follow will vary considerably according to the nature of the remedy, the severity of the condition, sensitivity, and response. Where *infrequent* repetition is required, this is indicated. With regard to the remaining remedies, dosage may vary from twice daily (12h) to twice weekly (or even less often) according to circumstances. The substitution of potencies less than that suggested is feasible.

(4) *Bilharzia 200* is essential in the treatment of both acute (at the onset) and chronic bilharzia, and is usually given at weekly intervals.

(5) *Medorrhinum 200* is often called for in chronic cases with advanced pelvic disease, covering as it does the fibrosis, granulomas, papillomas, and chronic urinary tract symptoms. This remedy should be repeated infrequently (not more often than once every 2 weeks).

251

(6) *Thuja 200*, or higher, is often indicated in these chronic cases, and, as with (5), should be repeated infrequently.

(7) *Carcinosin 200* should also be kept in mind in chronic cases, because of the tendency of the condition to ultimate in cancer of the bladder. It should be given in most chronic cases, but at infrequent intervals (not more often than once monthly).

(8) *Terebinthina 200*, or higher, is the most frequently indicated remedy for bilharziasis. The provings cover not only the symptoms of *S. haematobium*, but also those of *S. mansoni* and *S. japonicum*. It has the itching erythematous rash and urticaria of the initial stage, all the bowel, urinary, and even the respiratory symptoms and abdominal distention (ascites) of the advanced cases. Its use is well-known to old farmers in South Africa, who are less swayed by 'modern science'. They speak with reverence of the efficacy of a 'sip of turps' both as prophylactic and cure.

(9) *Chininum sulphuricum 200*, and *Cinchona officinalis 200* cover many of the symptoms and signs of the intestinal variety, and *Chininum arsenicosum 200* has helped many a chronic case where malaise, profound exhaustion and debility have been the presenting symptoms.

(10) *Antimonium tartaricum 200* is another magnificent remedy for bilharziasis, and is frequently indicated. It embraces both the symptoms of the genitourinary and intestinal varieties. The occurrence of drowsiness and debility strongly indicates the use of this remedy. It is always necessary in those patients, who are still seen, who have received in the past heroic doses of *Tartar Emetic* (Antimony Potassium Tartrate) for their bilharzia, and have never been well since. '*Never well since bilharzia*' also requires *Bilharzia 200*, once a week or once a fortnight.

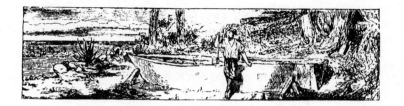

Section 22

TROPICAL SKIN ULCERS

Ulcers of the skin are extremely common in the tropics. It is important to distinguish between the diverse types, since their treatment varies considerably.

Tropical ulcer (Tropical phagedaenic ulcer)
The term *tropical (phagedaenic) ulcer* refers to a particular type of ulcer occurring in the tropics. The vast majority of these ulcers are found below the knee, and they are particularly common in tropical Africa, South America, and South-East Asia. Their exact causation is unknown, but it is believed that they may stem from secondary infection (by various bacteria) of insect bites or minor injuries to the skin. They are largely seen in rural land workers. The implication is that they may be preventable, if proper hygienic care is given to all breaks in the skin, no matter how minor.

Usually the disorder begins with a painful pimple (papule) or blister (often below the knee), which breaks down to form a painful ulcer. This grows rapidly over the course of a few weeks. The edges of the ulcer are red, slightly raised, swollen, and tender, but are not undermined. The ulcer not only extends in diameter, but also in depth, with the erosion of deeper tissues (there may be destruction of muscles, or even erosion of bone). Its smell is offensive, and its floor covered with pus. After several weeks, extension of the ulcer ceases, its ultimate diameter being in the range of 1–10cm (½-4in). Sometimes several ulcers are present.

Whilst some ulcers heal spontaneously, many remain unhealed for years. Important possible complications include: infection of bone (osteomyelitis), infection of joints (bacterial arthritis), tetanus, bacterial blood poisoning (septicaemia), secondary infection with diphtheria bacteria (see below under *Veld sore*), and cancer formation at the margin of the ulcer. In old ulcers, the floor is covered with dense fibrous tissue, and the potential for healing considerably diminished. Here, surgical excision and skin-grafting are clearly indicated as the only sensible recourse. It follows that early treatment of a tropical ulcer is of the utmost importance, of which the *local* measures (those applied directly to the ulcer) are the more significant:

(1) Superficial cleaning of the wound to eliminate slough (dead tissue), pus, and surface bacteria. The patient should be rested, and the ulcer irrigated with *hydrogen peroxide 1%*. A dressing soaked in *Rose Water* (*triple*) should then be applied. In order to prevent it drying out, it should be covered with any plastic sheeting available. The ulcer should be irrigated and dressed in this manner on a daily basis until the ulcer is clean (3–7 days). Credit for the notion that ulcers should be treated with wet dressings is to be given to the Swiss alchemical physician Paracelsus (Theophrastus Bombastus von Hohenheim, 1493–1541).

(2) The administration of internal homoeopathic remedies to promote both the immune response to bacteria in the tissues and local healing. Internal homoeopathic treatment should be started as early as possible, in conjunction with local cleansing. Commence with:

Mercurius solubilis 6 6h

(3) Improvement will be witnessed by a considerable reduction or absence of pain. Continue giving the remedy.

(4) Should the pain not improve within 7 days, change the internal prescription to:

Acidum nitricum 6 6h

(5) In indolent cases, substitute the following internal remedy:

Carbo vegetabilis 6 6h

(6) Once the ulcer is clean, and the pain considerably reduced, it is necessary to reinforce local healing. The irrigation and wet dressing technique described above is now abandoned, whilst the administration of the appropriate internal homoeopathic remedy is continued. It is now important to apply *non-adherent* dressings on a daily basis, and to cause as little damage as possible to the healing edge of the ulcer. Whilst paraffin gauze (tulle gras), or gauze soaked in coconut oil might be used, gauze generously impregnated with *Unguentum Calendulae* 5% is superior (*Cremor Calendulae* must not be used, since it will not prevent the dressing from sticking to the ulcer, which, when removed, will disturb areas of newly-formed skin).

(7) Should pus reappear in the base of the ulcer at any time during treatment with greasy dressings, then these must be abandoned in favour of the irrigation and wet dressing technique described in (1). Once the ulcer is clean, greasy dressings may be applied again.

(8) Treatment must be continued until complete healing is effected. Serious complications are usually preventable with early treatment, but should they arise, expert medical attention should be sought.

Buruli ulcer
This is a highly destructive ulcerative condition of the skin which has been described in Africa, South–East Asia, Papua New Guinea, and the Americas. It is caused by the bacterium *Mycobacterium ulcerans*, which is similar to that which causes tuberculosis. Unlike the latter, however, its mode of transmission is unknown, and thus no sensible advice can be given with regard to its avoidance.

Whereas it mainly involves the limbs (arms or legs), it may be found anywhere on the body, with the exception of the scalp. It begins as a firm painless nodule (or nodules), which may be slightly itchy. At this stage it may be confused with an insect bite, but careful inspection will fail to reveal a pit in the centre of the nodule characteristically produced by the latter. Neither is there any obvious inflammation. This nodule may then grow either rapidly over the course of several weeks, or more slowly for several months. Early recognition with surgical excision at this stage will result in a complete cure. Usually, however, it goes unrecognised, and proceeds to ulceration, which may progress with great rapidity, causing great destruction of skin tissue. This condition is readily distinguished from *tropical (phagedaenic) ulcer* (see above), on the basis of its clinical presentation: it is painless, and the edges of the ulcer are undermined (a tropical ulcer is painful, and the edges are not undermined). Satellite ulcers may be present, which communicate with the main ulcer by channels running under the skin. After the initial phase of rapid progression, the ulcer has a tendency to heal spontaneously over months or years, accompanied by considerable scarring and deformity of the tissues. Confirmation of the diagnosis may be made by bacteriological analysis of infected tissue.

Apart from attempting to eliminate the infection, surgical expertise is required to restore the integrity of the skin. Local treatment with antiseptics may be helpful. Freshly prepared *silver nitrate solution (Lotio Argenti Nitratis) 0.5%* is effective. Wet dressings of *Chelidonium majus* lotion may be tried for their anti-mycobacterial effect (*Chelidonium majus ø 1 part + clean water 9 parts*). Orthodox drugs, given by mouth, are also available. Homoeopathically, the internal remedy *Bacillinum*, given high and infrequently, under the guidance of an homoeopathic practitioner, may be helpful.

Veld sore (Veldt/Desert sore)
This is essentially *diphtheria* of the skin (see also *Section 3*). It usually occurs on the leg, but may occur elsewhere, such as the arm, or areas where the clothing has been rubbing. Poor hygiene, especially in the tropics or subtropics, leads to the infection of even minor injuries of the skin. The initial presentation is a small, painful blister (vesicle) filled with

straw-coloured fluid. On bursting, this becomes an ulcer. This ulcer is usually solitary, circular, and punched-out in appearance, with undermined, thickened, dusky blue margins. The base is covered with grey debris, beneath which may be found an adherent membrane of slough. The ulcer may persist for many months before healing spontaneously. The ulcer itself, however, is not the main problem. Far more important is the fact that the infecting diphtheria bacteria produce a potent toxin which affects the nervous system. The initial symptoms are numbness, coldness of the extremities, and blurred vision. Later there appear incoordination of movement, paralysis of the throat, and weakness of wrists (wrist drop) and ankles (ankle drop). The initial local paralysis is related to the site of the ulcer. More serious paralyses may follow, and death may ensue.

The combination of the characteristic appearance of the ulcer, with its punched-out margins and adherent slough, and the occurrence of paralysis is virtually diagnostic of Veld sore, even in the absence of bacteriological analysis of the tissue. In view of its serious potential, urgent medical advice should be sought, where possible. Homoeopathic treatment includes:

(1) The regular application of wet dressings of *Hydrastis lotion* to the ulcer (*Hydrastis ø 1 part + clean water 9 parts*).

(2) Additionally, the following two internal remedies may be given in combination *6h*:
    (a) *Kali bichromicum 6*
    (b) *Causticum 30*

(3) Additionally, where available, give internally:

Diphtherinum 30 12h

Dracontiasis (Dracunculiasis/Guinea worm infection)
About 10 million people are infected with the *Guinea worm (Dracunculus medinensis)*. It is found in West and central Africa (Cameroon to Mauritania, Uganda, southern Sudan), Saudi Arabia, Yemen, Iran, Turkestan, Brazil and the Indian subcontinent. According to area, up to 60% of the resident population may be so afflicted.

The infection is acquired by *swallowing* water containing

certain 'water fleas' (*Cyclops*), which harbour the immature (larval) forms of the worm. These larvae then penetrate the gut, and mature in the tissues. The male worm causes no immediate problem to its human host, and dies immediately after mating with a female. The pregnant female, which may attain a length of 1 metre (3ft) or more, gradually moves towards the surface of the body, reaching the latter approximately 9–14 months after initial infection. The first signs of disease appear as the head of the worm approaches the inner surface of the skin. The local symptoms include: redness, tenderness, burning and itching. Fever and urticaria (nettle-rash/hives) also occur. Less commonly, there are: diarrhoea, vomiting, wheezing, and fainting. The head of the worm produces a blister on the skin, which spontaneously ruptures, with the relief of general symptoms. A painful ulcer is produced, usually on the leg or foot (occasionally elsewhere), at the centre of which may be seen a pearly loop (the uterus of the worm). Whenever the ulcer comes in contact with water, larval worms are discharged, appearing as a milky fluid, which are then consumed by water fleas. In some cases, multiple ulcers are present. Complications, which are by no means uncommon, include: abscess formation, bacterial blood poisoning (septicaemia), arthritis (due to the worm entering a joint), and tetanus. Some septic complications may stem from inept attempts to remove the worm (see below).

Even without treatment many ulcers will resolve spontaneously within 6 weeks, with the worm dying in the tissues and becoming calcified. The treatment described below is only justified if it can be carried out competently and aseptically (hygienically). Otherwise, it is better to leave things alone until medical expertise is available.

The object of treatment is to shorten the period of disability, and reduce the likelihood of complications. The worm is removed by the method described by the Greek physician Hippocrates, with some minor modern improvements. Each day, for several days, the foot (or leg) is immersed in water for 30 minutes. This is to empty the extensive uterus of the worm. For ulcers in other parts of the body, wet compresses should be applied for a similar time.

The uterus is empty when no more milky fluid (the larvae) is discharged. The worm will now be more apparent at the centre of the ulcer, having slightly emerged, and should be grasped with forceps, and pulled out a little further. The worm must be secured to a thin, round, sterilized stick (a few millimetres in diameter) by means of thread, or by fixing it in a cleft cut into one end of the wood. Gentle traction is then applied by rolling the worm around the stick, stopping immediately when resistance is felt. The use of excessive force will rupture the worm, and severe inflammation of the tissues may follow. This procedure must be repeated once daily, until the worm is completely removed, which may take 14 days or more. The administration of the following internal homoeopathic remedy may hasten removal of the worm:

> *Silicea 6 6h*

Other than for periods of water immersion, wet compresses, or traction, it is most important to protect the ulcer with clean dressings to prevent secondary infection. These may be saturated with *Rose Water (triple)* for its antiseptic properties.

Guinea worm infection may be *prevented* by the filtration of water through two layers of shirt material, which effectively removes the water fleas. Alternatively, the water may be boiled. Certain places are particularly notorious with regard to contamination, notably the step-wells of India, where the water-carriers frequently develop Guinea worm ulcers on their backs. Running water is less likely to be hazardous than that from a well.

Cutaneous leishmaniasis

This disease is one of the most significant causes of ulcerative and disfiguring skin lesions in the World, and travellers may acquire it with great ease. The causative microorganisms, *Leishmania*, of which there are various types, are protozoan parasites transmitted by the bites of the females of certain species of *sandfly*. Various animals (such as dogs, foxes, jackals, and gerbils) act as reservoirs of infection.

The prevention of sandfly bites is of the utmost importance. In addition to the general measures stated in *Section*

14, additional preventative steps will be necessary based upon the known characteristics of the sandfly, in terms of size and behaviour. The following points are worthy of note:

(1) Sandflies are light yellow or grey flies with long, slender legs, giving them the appearance of standing on stilts. Being usually no more than 2–3mm (1/8th in) long, they will readily pass through standard mosquito netting. Impregnation of the latter with insecticide will improve its performance, and may be preferable to the use of finer sandfly netting, which is so closely woven that it may be unbearable at night in hot climates.

(2) Sandflies do not fly very high (usually less than 60cm/ 2ft). You are, therefore, less likely to be bitten if you travel by horse or camel, and sleep on the first floor, or above, in any building. If the building has a single storey, sleep on the roof.

(3) Sandflies have a short range of flight, and seldom travel more than 200m (220yds) from their breeding sites. These include: piles of rubble, cracks in walls, caves, outside privies, termite mounds, and other dark and damp places. Many of these are recognisable and avoidable. Avoid camping near gerbil colonies in the Middle East, and do not sleep in villages where many of the residents exhibit irregular scarring on their faces.

(4) Sandflies do not only bite at night. They are particularly aggressive at dawn and dusk, and you should avoid going for walks at these times.

We shall now discuss the three main varieties of cutaneous leishmaniasis:

(a) Old World cutaneous leishmaniasis
(b) New World (American) cutaneous leishmaniasis
(c) New World (American) mucocutaneous leishmaniasis

[another form of leishmaniasis, known as *kala azar (visceral leishmaniasis)*, and mainly a disease of internal organs, is discussed in *Section 26*]

Old World cutaneous leishmaniasis (Oriental sore)

This occurs in many areas of the tropics and subtropics, the Mediterranean, the Middle East, North Africa, and Asiatic Russia. The clinical disease produced varies with the particular species of parasite involved. The *urban* variety (*Leishmania tropica*), where the dog is the natural reservoir of infection, is often found in big cities, such as Baghdad, Aleppo, Damascus, Tehran, and Delhi, and also in the Spanish Costa del Sol, southern France and Italy, Majorca, and the Greek Islands. The *rural* form (*Leishmania major*) is not uncommon in the semi-desert areas of Iran, Iraq, northeastern Saudi Arabia, Jordan, and Israel, and here the natural reservoir is the gerbil. It is also found in Afghanistan, the southern part of the former USSR, and Africa.

The infection is generally limited to the area of the sandfly bite (often the face or arm), first signs of which may appear from several days to several months after the event. The typical *urban* lesion is a single, dry nodule on the skin, which ulcerates slowly or not at all, which tends to be painless in the absence of secondary bacterial infection, and which heals in a year or more, with significant scarring. In contrast, the typical *rural* form, after the development of an initial large nodule (2cm/1in in diameter), rapidly progresses to the production of multiple, wet, ulcerating sores with crusting, which, however, tend to heal more rapidly, but with greater scarring. Yet another variety is produced by *L. aethiopica*, found in the Ethiopian and Kenyan highlands, and South-West Africa, where the natural animal reservoirs include the rock hyrax, tree hyrax, and giant rat. Here, the lesions usually resemble those of the urban variety described above, but spontaneous healing is slow, and they may persist for several years. An uncommon complication of this infection is the generation of multiple non-ulcerative lesions over the entire body, resembling *lepromatous leprosy* (see *Section 23*).

The diagnosis of the disease is confirmed by taking scrapings, or aspirating fluid, from the cleaned edge of the ulcer, and not from any normal discharge, since this is invariably free of the offending parasite.

In general, the lesions of Old World cutaneous

leishmaniasis heal spontaneously, without any special treatment, and immunity to further infections is conferred. Scarring is the worst problem, which may either produce cosmetic disfigurement, or, if it occurs in the region of a joint, such as the wrist, limitation of movement. Secondary infection of ulcerated areas will be prevented by careful hygiene, including regular irrigation with *Rose Water (triple)*. Other treatments, including the use of orthodox antiparasitic drugs, may be used to shorten the course and intensity of the disorder, and to minimise the production of scar tissue. Homoeopathically, a *nosode* (a remedy made from infected material), corresponding to the appropriate species of *Leishmania*, may be used throughout the course of the disorder. For example, in the case of urban leishmaniasis:

> *Leishmania tropica ('canis') 30 once weekly*

Additionally, once the healing phase has set in, the following may be used to reduce scarring:

(1) Internally, give:

> *Thiosinaminum 6 12h*

(2) Externally, apply the following cream *12h*:

> *Cremoris Graphitum 8x*   *30g*
> *d-Alpha Tocopheryl Acetati*   *600IU*

New World cutaneous leishmaniasis
In the Americas, cutaneous leishmaniasis is endemic from Argentina through to Mexico (Yucatan), and is found, albeit rarely, in the southern USA. Animal reservoirs of infection include: rodents, marmosets, sloths, and anteaters. Diagnosis is established through scrapings, biopsy, or aspirated tissue fluid. The majority of New World lesions are ulcers, but nodules and wart-like lesions also occur. In the Yucatan and Central America, *L. mexicana mexicana* is the cause of *chiclero's ulcer*, a destructive ulcerative condition of the cartilage of the ear, common in those who gather the latex used in the production of chewing gum. *L. mexicana amazonensis* and *L. mexicana pifanoi* may produce multiple skin lesions, rather like those of *L. aethiopica* (see above), which

resemble lepromatous leprosy. Of even greater, importance, disease produced by *L. braziliensis braziliensis* may progress to the serious condition known as *mucocutaneous leishmaniasis*, described separately below.

New World mucocutaneous leishmaniasis (Espundia)

L. braziliensis braziliensis is the cause of severe destructive lesions of the mouth and nose in lowland forest areas of South America, and Central America, North to Belize. This is the disease known as mucocutaneous leishmaniasis or *espundia*. In that it is essentially a rural disorder, it will be of little concern to those who stay within the bounds of cities. The vector is an aggressive sandfly which will attack even *in the day*, if the sky is overcast. The animal reservoir is not known for certain, but may be the dog or the horse. More rarely, espundia is caused by *L. braziliensis panamensis*, found in Panama and probably elsewhere in South America, where the reservoir of infection is the sloth.

Unfortunately for the clinician, the initial lesions produced are virtually indistinguishable from those of the more benign varieties of New World cutaneous leishmaniasis (see above). After an initial incubation period of at least 15 days, the initial lesion, which may be single or multiple, appears on exposed skin, usually the front of the lower third of the leg. This is an itchy or painful lump, which becomes nodular, and then ulcerates or becomes wart-like. This lesion then slowly heals over a period of 3–12 months, with the production of scar tissue. In up to 80% of patients, subsequent lesions then appear in the nose. They may appear concurrently with the initial lesion, shortly after healing, or there may be a considerable delay in their development of 2–20 years. The front of the internal dividing septum of the nose is generally the first area involved. There may be blockage, catarrh, pain, or bleeding. The disease may then progress to involve the rest of the nose, the palate, the mouth, the throat, and the larynx. Ulcers and polyps are found on examination, along with considerable destruction of tissues, producing hideous deformities if allowed to progress. Secondary bacterial infection is not uncommon. The whole appearance of an established case resembles cancerous destruction of the face, with which it may be confused, but from which it may be distinguished by means of biopsy.

Treatment of New World cutaneous and mucocutaneous leishmaniasis

Whilst it is true to say that most nodules or ulcers will heal spontaneously, even in the absence of any treatment other than the prevention of secondary bacterial infection, there is, however, apart from the obvious problem of scarring, a decided risk of the development of espundia in some. In the absence of special tests, it is probably wise, therefore, to treat all cases in endemic espundia areas at the earliest possible opportunity. Any nodules, wart-like lesions, or ulcers apparently contracted by a visit to such an area should not be disregarded, and the advice of an experienced physician should be sought. Orthodox drugs are available, but homoeopathy may make valuable contributions; this especially so in the case of established severe espundia, where failure rates to orthodox medicine are high. The following comments are particularly directed to those medical or paramedical persons with some homoeopathic experience:

(1) In all cases, the internal administration of a *nosode* prepared from diseased tissue, and matching the particular species of *Leishmania* involved in the particular case, may be given in the *30th* potency, or higher, once weekly. Where microbiological confirmation of the species is unavailable, scrapings or aspirated fluid from the edge of an ulcer, or biopsy material, may be sent (in 80–90% alcohol) to the homoeopathic pharmacist for potentization (preparation of the homoeopathic remedy). Alternatively, a mixed nosode, corresponding to several strains of *Leishmania*, including especially *L. braziliensis braziliensis*, may be given similarly.

(2) Additionally, in established cases of espundia, the internal remedy *Medorrhinum 200*, given no more frequently than once every two weeks, should be administered, especially with polyp formation. Also *Thuja 200* should be considered, with similar infrequent repetition.

(3) Additionally, in established cases of espundia, with

erosion and destruction of the nasal septum, any of the following internal remedies, may be considered:

    (a) *Aurum metallicum 6 6–12h*
    (b) *Kali bichromicum 6 6–12h*
    (c) *Hippozaeninum 30 once weekly*

Other causes of chronic tropical skin ulcers

    (1) Tuberculosis (see Section 23).
    (2) Adult sickle cell disease (rare in Africa).
    (3) Trophic ulcer in leprosy (see Section 23).
    (4) Tertiary syphilis (gumma).

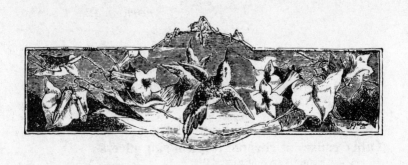

SOME INFAMOUS BACTERIA

Despite the advent of the antibiotic, bacterial disease is still a major cause of disability and mortality.

Typhoid (Enteric fever)
The two most common causes of *fever* in those returning from visits to hot climates are malaria (see *Section 20*) and typhoid. Typhoid, transmitted via the ingestion of contaminated food or water, and thus a disease of poor hygiene, is distributed world-wide, but is most common in the tropics and subtropics. The causative organism is *Salmonella typhi*. With regard to its prevention, consult *Sections 3* and *10* of this manual. It is to be noted that those with low stomach acidity (eg persons taking antacid drugs) are more prone to the contraction of this disease.

The incubation period is generally 8–18 days; although it may be as short as 3, or as long as 60 days. Typically, the following stages of the disease are described:

(1) *The first week*. Malaise (feeling unwell), severe headache, lack of appetite, sore throat, coated tongue, inflamed

throat, dry cough, nosebleed, vague abdominal pains, and *constipation*. At this stage it might be confused with common *influenza*. However, the characteristics of the fever may be quite different. The temperature may rise in the first week in a step-like fashion to 39–40°C (102–104°F), yet the pulse may remain unusually *slow*. In most fevers, the pulse rate normally increases by 18 beats/minute for every 1°C rise in temperature (32 beats/minute per 1°F). In typhoid, however, the pulse may be 20–40 beats/minute slower than that which would be normally expected. Even at 40°C, the pulse rate may be less than 100 beats/minute (relative slowness of the pulse is also seen in yellow fever, dengue, typhus, and sandfly fever).

(2) *The second week*. The temperature remains elevated, but the pulse rate gains. The abdominal symptoms become more obvious, and there may be pain and tenderness in the right side of the lower abdomen (the 'appendix area'). The liver and spleen become enlarged, and are palpable by the experienced. At 7–10 days, pale rose-coloured spots appear, approximately 2–5mm in diameter, which are slightly raised and fade on pressure. In most cases they are found on the trunk, and vary in number from 2 or 3 to many.

(3) *The end of the second week into the third week*. This is the most dangerous phase of the disease. In 25% of cases, constipation gives place to a diarrhoea resembling 'pea soup'. There may be confusion, immobility (with a blank stare, though rousable), agitation, disorientation, or delirium. The headache is severe, and neck stiffness may occur (resembling meningitis). Intestinal bleeding and per-foration of the bowel may follow, with fatal consequences. Intestinal perforation occurs in 3–4% of cases, and intestinal bleeding in 2–8%.

Thus, have been described the features of 'typical' typhoid; and life would be grand for the clinician if all cases presented similarly, for, even without special tests (including blood tests), the diagnosis would be obvious. Regrettably, however, more cases are 'atypical' rather than 'typical':

(a) In the first week, the temperature does not necessarily rise in steps. It may exhibit a fulminating rise in the first day or two, and, after a plateau, remits in the mornings, with a gradual decline to normality. In other cases, the fever may be intermittent (periodic), resembling *malaria*, and in others it may be low.

(b) The relative deficiency of the pulse rate described above is very typical of typhoid, but may not be apparent.

(c) Rose spots may be absent, and are seldom seen in Negroes.

(d) In young children, it may present with severe diarrhoea, vomiting, dehydration, stiff neck, and convulsions.

(e) Mild tropical cases in children may present as simple diarrhoea.

(f) Jaundice, uncommon in adults, occurs in approximately 7% of children's cases.

(g) In the tropics, many patients, whilst exhibiting a fever, remain ambulant until there is a sudden onset of acute abdominal pain.

The possible complications of typhoid are numerous. Intestinal bleeding and perforation have already be mentioned. Others include: acute inflammation of the gallbladder, pneumonia, thrombosis (clotting) of the veins, haemolytic anaemia (destruction of red blood cells), meningitis (1% of cases), abscesses of the parotid salivary glands, hepatitis, inflammation of the heart (endocarditis), neuritis ('burning feet'), temporary nerve deafness, urinary infection, abscess of the spleen, acute arthritis, and inflammation of bones (osteomyelitis).

Even after recovery, approximately 10% of patients will continue to excrete typhoid bacteria in their faeces or urine for some months; 3% will excrete them for over 12 months, and these 'chronic carriers' represent a considerable danger to public health, especially if involved in the preparation of food or drink for others. Removal of the gallbladder, which may harbour the bacteria, is indicated in some cases.

Paratyphoid (Enteric Fever)

The organisms *Salmonella paratyphi A, B, and C* are capable of producing *paratyphoid*, an illness, or rather a group of illnesses, very similar to typhoid in many respects. The term *enteric fever* is used to describe disease produced by either *S. typhi* or *S. paratyphi*. Transmission of paratyphoid is generally via contaminated food. See also *Sections 3* and *10* with regard to prevention.

Paratyphoid A is found in the USA, eastern Europe, India, and the Far East. Paratyphoid B is found in Europe and North America. They differ from typhoid in that diarrhoea and vomiting often precede the graver aspects of the illness. Many minor cases occur, without serious complications.

Paratyphoid C, is found in eastern Europe, and is rife in Guyana. In this condition, involvement of the intestine (bleeding or perforation) is unusual, but the production of deep-seated abscesses is common.

Rose-coloured spots are more profuse in paratyphoid infections, especially with regard to Paratyphoid A.

Treatment of enteric fever (typhoid and paratyphoid)

In view of the potential for serious complications, early recognition and treatment are desirable. As I have implied, in view of the diversity of presenting symptoms, considerable medical expertise may be required to effect a correct diagnosis. In treatment, orthodox drugs are available, blood transfusion may be required for haemorrhage, intravenous fluids for dehydration, and surgery for intestinal perforation with peritonitis (inflammation of the abdominal cavity). Homoeopathy is, however, not without place in the treatment of enteric fever, and with regard to this matter the following observations and suggestions may be made:

(1) The internal homoeopathic treatment should begin at the earliest possible opportunity (preferably within the first 7 days of illness). Even if the case is 'atypical', but enteric fever is suspected as a possibility, due to symptoms or circumstances (eg a typhoid outbreak in the vicinity), then appropriate treatment should be instituted along the lines that follow.

(2) In both early 'typical' and suspected 'atypical' cases give:

Ipecacuanha 30 6h

This prescription should be given for 2 days, and no longer. Should cerebral symptoms develop (such as confusion, disorientation, immobility, agitation, or delirium), it must be abandoned in favour of that which follows.

(3) Following 2 days of *Ipecacuanha*, or less, if cerebral symptoms supervene, give in conjunction:

  (a) *Belladonna 30 one dose early morning, and another 6 hours later*

  (b) *Acidum muriaticum 6 one dose in the evening, about 6 hours after the second dose of the above*

This prescription may be continued on a daily basis until significant improvement has occurred (the development of serious complications will warrant other remedies).

(4) As an alternative, in early cases, instead of prescriptions (2) and (3), the following two remedies may be given in alternation (alternately), with a dosage interval of 4 hours:

  (a) *Baptisia 30*

  (b) *Gelsemium 30*

(5) Once significant improvement has occurred, any diarrhoea has stopped, and yet the patient has some debility, and dryness of the mouth and lips, abandon the above, and give for 2 days:

  Cinchona officinalis 30 6h

(6) Relapse may occur 5–14 days after apparent recovery, if initial treatment has been inadequate. Such relapse is usually less severe than the original attack. Repetition of the former treatment will generally be required.

(7) In cases of temporary nerve deafness, in order to accelerate recovery, give:

  Nux vomica 6 6h

(8) In cases of neuritis, with 'burning feet', give generous doses of *vitamin B complex* by mouth for several weeks.

Further indications for homoeopathic remedies in enteric fever

(a) Delirium: Belladonna, Gelsemium, Hyoscyamus, Stramonium.

(b) Bronchitis or pneumonia: Phosphorus and Bryonia, in alternation.

(c) Perforation and peritonitis: Aconite, given frequently.

(d) Intestinal haemorrhage: Acidum nitricum, Phosphorus, Lachesis, Hamamelis.
(e) Urinary symptoms: Terebinthina.
(f) Feeling bruised (complains of hardness of bed): Arnica.
(g) Pains in limbs and body, relieved by movement, and great restlessness: Rhus toxicodendron.

Plague (Black Death)

Plague, once the scourge of Europe and elsewhere, is no longer a disease of great concern to the average traveller. The infective microorganism, *Yersinia pestis*, is harboured by rodents, and mainly transmitted to humans by the bites of certain species of flea which live upon the latter. The greatest risk is during the warm, rather than hot, summer months. Transmission without fleas may also occur, by the handling of infected animals (alive or dead), and by droplet spread from a human sufferer (leading to pneumonic plague). It is highly contagious. Plague is currently endemic in the western USA, South America, Asia, and Africa. It is of greatest concern to hunters, naturalists, campers, and explorers, and may be prevented in the following ways:

(1) Avoid handling live or dead rodents (eg rats, chipmunks, marmots, rabbits, squirrels) in endemic plague areas.

(2) Use flea repellents for rural excursions, and insecticides in the domestic situation (see *Section 14*).

(3) Control rodents in the domestic area.

(4) Immunization for high-risk individuals, such as zoologists (see *Section 3*).

(5) Since infections sometimes occur via domestic pets in endemic areas, they should be regularly treated with anti-flea agents.

The classic form of the disease is *bubonic* plague. After an incubation period of 2–7 days there is a *sudden onset* of high fever, severe headache, chill (shivering), and muscular pains. Both pulse and breathing become rapid. Initial mental dullness gives way to a state of anxiety, an intense facial expression of which is characteristic of the illness. The tongue is coated, the eyes and face red, and nausea, vomiting, constipation, and scanty urine are fairly typical. Delirium, coma, or convulsions (children) may occur. In 75% of cases enlarged lymph-glands, termed *buboes*, appear. They generally appear 2–5 days after the onset of the illness, preceded by local pain. They may be situated in the groin (65–75%), the arm-pit (15–20%), the neck (5–10%), or elsewhere. They are extremely painful, and, when fully developed, may achieve the size of a hen's egg. In fatal cases they remain hard, but in others they proceed to abscess formation. Incision of these abscesses is hazardous, in that it may cause infection of the blood (septicaemia). At the site of inoculation, a pustule (small pus-filled blister) is occasionally observed. Sometimes a skin rash resembling smallpox occurs.

Whilst pneumonia may occur as a complication of bubonic plague, a *primary pneumonic* variety of plague does occur. which presents as a fulminating, and usually fatal, pneumonia. In *primary septicaemic* plague, the bacteria spread rapidly throughout the body, and the patient usually dies within 3 days, before any buboes develop. Haemorrhages are not uncommon in this form. *Pestis minor*, as the name would suggest, is the most benign form of the disease. The patient is ambulant, there is little fever, and there is a single bubo in one groin, one side of the neck, or one arm-pit. These either gradually disappear, or proceed to abscess formation. The dangers of incision have been mentioned.

Bacteriological studies are helpful in the confirmation of the disease, but, where suspected, treatment must not be delayed whilst awaiting the results of the former. The mortality rate in untreated cases is 60–95%. Orthodox treatment is available, and homoeopathy may be useful. The following internal remedy should be given in early cases, until medical assistance can be obtained:

Baptisia 30 1h

Other homoeopathic remedies in plague

Cellulitis of neck: Apis mellifica (ø-low).
Meningism: Apis mellifica (ø-low).
Delirium (incoherence, picking at bed-clothes): Hyoscyamus.
Delirium (violent): Stramonium.

Later plague with bubonic abscesses: Mercurius cyanatus.
Primary septicaemia: Naja.
Pneumonic plague: Phosphorus.
Haemorrhage: Crotalus horridus (6x-12x).
Convalescence: Silicea.

Tularaemia (Rabbit/Lemming/Deer-fly fever)

This plague-like disease, caused by the bacterium *Francisella tularensis*, and essentially an infection of wild rodents, is transmissible to man via the handling of infected animals (alive or dead), the bites of arthropods (ticks, deer-flies, mosquitoes, and others), and the ingestion of contaminated water. The main animal reservoirs in North America are the jack rabbit, and hare; in Scandinavia, the lemming and hare; in Central Europe and France, the rabbit and hare; in the former USSR, the water rat, and the muskrat. The disease also occurs in Turkey and Japan.

After an incubation period of 2–10 days, there is a sudden onset of fever, nausea, and headache. At the site of inoculation, a red papule (pimple) appears, which develops into a pustule (small pus-filled blister), and then becomes a punched-out ulcer. This local lesion is generally on an extremity, but may occur in the eye. The regional lymph-glands become enlarged, and may undergo abscess formation. Pneumonia may occur. Where the organism has been ingested, rather than inoculated, a typhoid-like form of disease is produced (see above, under *typhoid*). In any type of the disease, enlargement of the spleen, generalized pains, skin rashes, and prostration may occur.

The diagnosis is confirmed by blood tests, and the mortality rate in untreated cases is approximately 7%. Treatment may be given with orthodox drugs. Homoeopathic treatment may be administered along the lines suggested for plague, or typhoid (see above), according to type.

Relapsing fever (Famine/Tick/Tick-bite/Recurrent fever)

This disease, caused by various species of the spirochaete (spiral bacterium) *Borrelia*, is found in many parts of the World. It is transmitted by either lice or ticks. Louse-borne relapsing fever is essentially a disease associated with squalor, poverty, and malnutrition, and may be found in virtually any area where such conditions prevail. Tick-borne relapsing fever, in which rodents act as a natural reservoir of infection, is prevalent in the southern USA, Central and South America, Africa (South of the Sahara), the Mediterranean (including Spain, Cyprus, Israel, and North Africa), the near East, and the southern section of the former USSR; it is not to be found in Australia. In North Africa, beware of the caves, which commonly harbour ticks. For general measures of prevention see *Sections 14 and 16*.

The incubation period is 1–14 days. There is a sudden onset of fever, chills (shivering), severe headache, joint pains, nausea, and vomiting. The attack terminates abruptly on the third or fourth day. Typically, the attack returns after 7–14 days, often in a milder form, and again rapid in onset and termination. 3–10 relapses may occur before the illness finally disappears. Complications include: enlargement of the spleen (45%), enlargement of the liver (11%), jaundice, bronchitis, pneumonia, paralysis (including facial paralysis), and inflammation of the eye (iritis, iridocyclitis). The overall mortality is approximately 5%.

The initial attack may be confused with malaria (see *Section 20*), but the interval between this and subsequent attacks is characteristically longer in relapsing fever. Microbiological studies, where available, are useful. Treatment should be started as soon as possible, even in the absence of the latter, where relapsing fever is suspected. Orthodox drug therapy is available. Homoeopathically, commence treatment with the following two remedies, given *in alternation (alternately) every 2 hours*:

(1) Bryonia 30
(2) Rhus toxicodendron 30

Other homoeopathic remedies in relapsing fever

Severe pains in limbs and back: Eupatorium perfoliatum.
Enlargement of liver and spleen: Mercurius solubilis.
Relapsed cases with great prostration and thirst for sips: Arsenicum album.

Delirium: Hyoscyamus.
Sudden collapse with coldness of body: Veratrum album.

Brucellosis (Undulant/Malta/Rio Grande/ Mediterranean fever)

Brucellosis, caused by the bacteria *Brucella abortus* and *Brucella melitensis*, is of relevance to the traveller in that it may be contracted by drinking unpasteurised milk or milk-products. *B. abortus* is mainly found in cows' milk, and *B. melitensis* in goats' milk. The goats' milk cheese of Malta has been a particularly notorious source of infection.

The incubation period is usually 1–3 weeks, but may be several months. The onset may be sudden (acute) or insidious. The acute form, which may last for several weeks, consists of fever (with late afternoon spikes of up to 40°C/104°F), chills (shivering), profuse and sour-smelling sweat, severe joint pains (one or more larger joints), and inflammation of the testicle (orchitis or epididymitis). Following the acute phase, there may evolve a chronic stage, which may last for years.

As either a sequel to the acute illness, or developing insidiously, the chronic phase is characterised by: weakness, loss of weight, exhaustion, sweating, fever, enlargement of the lymph glands and spleen (50%), and sometimes enlargement of the liver. Various types of fever have been described with regard to brucellosis, but the most characteristic is the *undulant* form, which may persist for many months. Typically, there is a ladder-like rise for 7–10 days up to 40°C (104°F), followed by a gradual fall to normal over a period of 7–10 days. The phase of normal temperature, lasting several days, is immediately followed by a recurrence of fever of the pattern described.

Some cases may be confused with *typhoid* (see above), but the temperature chart will assist in differentiation. In brucellosis the daily peak of the fever is late morning or afternoon, whereas in typhoid it is towards the night. A chronic form of brucellosis, found in East Africa, with gross enlargement of spleen and liver, may be confused with *kala azar* (see *Section 26*). Special investigations may be necessary to confirm the diagnosis.

Generally, brucellosis will burn itself out, and 50% of sufferers will recover spontaneously within 12 months. The mortality rate in untreated cases is about 2%, death usually resulting from infection of the heart (endocarditis). Orthodox treatment is available, but homoeopathy is especially useful, particularly in chronic cases. Either solely, or as an adjunct to other indicated homoeopathic remedies, the following should be given routinely in all cases:

Brucella abortus et melitensis nosode 30 once weekly

Other homoeopathic remedies in brucellosis
Baptisia, Gelsemium, Eupatorium perfoliatum, and Rhus toxicodendron have been suggested, according to their particular indications. In addition, for late afternoon fever with sour sweat, consider Lycopodium. For orchitis or epididymitis, consider either Pulsatilla or Rhododendron.

Leptospirosis
This disease, or rather, group of diseases, of world-wide distribution, is contracted by the contact of skin abrasions and wounds with infected rats' urine. The infective organisms are various species of spirochaete (spiral bacteria) of the genus *Leptospira*. With regard to travellers, the more important variety of this disease will be that found in South-East Asia, where, in Malaysia, it accounts for over 10% of rural hospital admissions for *fever*. It is also common in rural Thailand. Those who travel along the banks of rivers or streams, or venture into rice fields will be at greatest risk. The causative organism, *Leptospira interrogans*, unlike its European and American relatives, *seldom causes jaundice*. The illness presents with an abrupt and high fever (39–40°C/102.2–104°F), congestion of the face, severe headache, chills (shivering), abdominal pain and tenderness, and vomiting. Characteristically, the muscles, especially those of the calf, are intensely painful and tender, and the degree of prostration, which is profound, is totally out of proportion to the observable vital signs (blood pressure, pulse, etc.). Complications include: haemorrhages (eg from the lungs), and kidney failure. Special tests may be required to confirm the diagnosis, and orthodox treatment is available. Homoeo-

pathically, treatment may begin with the following internal remedy:

Arsenicum album 6 2h

Bartonellosis (Oroya fever/Carrion's disease/Verruga Peruviana)

This disease, caused by the bacterium *Bartonella bacilliformis* and spread by the bites of *sandflies*, is endemic on the steep valley slopes of Colombia, Ecuador, and Peru. With regard to general preventative measures, see *Sections 14* and *22*.

The incubation period is about 2–3 weeks. The onset of the disease is marked by fever, muscle and joint pains, and tender enlargement of the lymph glands. Haemolytic anaemia, due to disruption of the red blood cells, and enlargement of the liver and spleen may occur. This stage of the illness, which is called *Oroya fever (Carrion's Disease)*, may last 4–8 weeks, and carries a mortality rate of up to 40%, if untreated. The bacterium may be identified in the red blood cells.

The second stage of the disease, which is called *verruga peruviana (or peruana)* and occurs about 16 weeks after infection, may develop even in the absence of an attack of Oroya fever. Multiple vascular nodules (composed of small blood vessels), either flat or pedunculated (on stalks), appear on the skin, particularly on the face and limbs, with the largest ones, about the size of a pigeon's egg, being located on the knee or elbow. Others may develop in the upper part of the digestive system or female genitalia, and bleed. Untreated, they persist for several years.

Whilst orthodox therapy is available for Oroya fever, there is no known conventional treatment for verruga peruviana. With respect to the latter, amongst other internal remedies, the following may be tried:

Thuja 6 12h

Leprosy

This disease, endemic in the hotter parts of the World and caused by the bacterium *Mycobacterium leprae*, will be of little direct concern to the average traveller. Whilst it is spread by droplets from the nose or mouth of a sufferer, it is of extremely low infectivity, and seldom occurs in those who have but a fleeting contact with such a person.

The symptoms that develop are slow in progression, and vary considerably, in accord with the level of natural resistance. We shall confine ourselves to the main manifestations of the disease:

(1) Loss of feeling in the hands, then the feet. The patient may burn himself without realising. Skin ulcers, which are painless, develop as the result of trauma to hands or feet.

(2) Variable skin signs. Pale, flat spots, or rings resembling ringworm, with *loss of feeling* in the centre. Multiple nodular skin lesions (lepromatous leprosy). Ulcers (see above).

(3) Shortening of fingers and toes.

(4) Loss of eyebrows (first the outer part, then in entirety).

(5) Blindness.

With regard to treatment, in addition to advising the patient on the care of injuries to the skin of hands and feet, both orthodox and homoeopathic therapies are available.

Homoeopathic treatment of leprosy
Bacillinum, given high and infrequently, may be of value in any form of the disease. Others to be considered include: Arsenicum album, Alumina, Antimonium tartaricum, Anacardium, Sepia, Silicea, and Sulphur.

Some other important bacterial diseases
A few other bacterial diseases are worthy of mention, in view of the distinct possibility of coming in contact with them by virtue of itinerary or circumstances, the homoeopathic treatments for which are outside the province of the text. Urgent medical assistance is advisable in all cases.

Tuberculosis (TB) is a serious and contagious disease, not uncommon in developing and tropical countries. The most important form of the disease is that which affects the lungs, which is contracted by inhaling droplets of sputum from a sufferer. The most frequent signs of pulmonary TB are: chronic cough (worse on waking), fever in the afternoon, night sweats, pain in the chest or upper back, chronic weight loss, and increasing weakness. In more advanced cases, the skin becomes pale and waxy, blood is coughed up, and the voice may become hoarse, the latter being a most serious symptom. Tuberculosis of the skin causes a variety of painless lesions: skin ulcers, large wart-like lesions, or disfiguring tumours. Tuberculosis of the lymph glands of the neck, which may be contracted by the consumption of unpasteurised milk or milk-products, produces painless enlargement of those structures, with a tendency to abscess formation and discharge. Tuberculosis may produce meningitis, especially in young children, but its development (over days or weeks) is slower that of meningococcal meningitis (see below).

The prevention and principal zones of risk of *meningococcal meningitis* have been discussed in *Section 3*. Symptoms include: fever, severe headache, *stiff neck*, vomiting, somnolence, convulsions, and coma. A blotchy skin rash may occur in advance of more serious symptoms, and death may occur within a few hours. Viral meningitis produces a similar symptomatic picture, but with the absence of the characteristic rash.

Legionnaires' disease is a bacterial pneumonia, more commonly found in smokers, persons with chronic lung disorders, and those with defective immune systems. The infection is mainly acquired via inadequately maintained airconditioning plant in offices or hotels, or from showers and jacuzzis in apartments and hotels which have been poorly maintained, or little used. Symptoms include: cough, chest pain, fever, diarrhoea, vomiting, confusion, and loss of balance.

Melioidosis is mainly to be found in Malaysia, Vietnam, Sri Lanka, and Burma. Infection is probably acquired by contact of skin abrasions or wounds with moist soil or surface water that breeds the infective bacterium *Pseudomonas pseudomallei*. The disease presents itself in a number of different ways, which include: a single and persistent abscess under the skin; a short fever, with spontaneous resolution; a high fever, with chills (shivering), diarrhoea, and sometimes abscess formation; pneumonia; or chronic inflammation of the lymph glands, bones, joints, or liver.

A variety of bacterial *venereal* diseases, including syphilis and gonorrhoea, may be contracted by the indulgent. Sexual association with unknown or overtly promiscuous partners will place the traveller at great risk. It is now understood that the contraction of such diseases renders the sufferer all the more likely to contract AIDS. Those who must indulge in risky practices, should always have condoms at the ready.

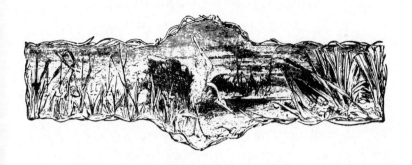

Section 24

VARIOUS VIRUSES

Whereas orthodox medicine is extremely limited in its armamentarium of antiviral drugs, homoeopathy, by stimulating the defensive (immune) systems of the body, is not so fettered. Special tests may be available to confirm the diagnosis of each disease described, but in some situations such availability will be limited or absent, and a thorough appraisal of clinical signs will be the sole or main method by which identification of the disorder is achieved, and the appropriate treatment determined.

Dengue (Breakbone/Dandy/Dengue fever)

Dengue is caused by a virus transmitted from man to man by the bites of various species of *Aeges* mosquito. It is endemic in Africa, the Pacific region, South-East Asia, and the Americas; and recurrent epidemics occur in the Caribbean. With regard to prevention, see *Sections 3* and *14*.

The incubation period is generally 5–8 days, but may be as short as 2½ or as long as 15 days. Headache, stiffness, backache, lack of appetite, weakness, chilliness, and a rash in some, may occur 6–12 hours before the onset of fever. However, in approximately 50% of cases, the onset is *sudden*, with an abrupt rise in temperature, flushed face, severe pain in muscles and joints (as though the bones were being broken), intense pain in the forehead and behind the eyes (which are congested), backache, and chilliness. Unlike *benign malaria*, shaking chills are rare. The fever generally persists for 5–6 days, before abating. In some cases, the temperature chart is of the *saddleback (diphasic)* type, where the temperature returns to normal at about 3–4 days, at which level it remains for 1 day, only to be followed by a recrudescence of fever (a similar diphasic effect may occur in yellow fever). As with typhoid, typhus, yellow fever, and sandfly fever, the pulse may be *slower* than that which might be expected from the level of the temperature, this phenomenon being especially marked in the second (recrudescent) phase of saddleback fever. The lymph-glands become enlarged in many cases, and the spleen only rarely. A rash often appears around days 3–5, consisting of slightly raised, red patches, fading on pressure, first appearing on the torso, and eventually spreading to the limbs and chest. The fever generally abates a few days after its appearance, with a return to normality. Even without treatment, the majority of cases recover spontaneously, and the mortality rate is extremely low.

However, in some cases, the more serious disease known as *dengue haemorrhagic fever* may ensue. Whilst the immunity conferred by an attack of dengue is short-lived (1–2 years), individuals still possessing antibodies from a previous attack, when re-infected with a different strain of dengue virus, may produce a more devastating disease reaction. Such a reaction is most common in children aged between 3 and 6, but adults are not exempt. Whereas the initial 3–4 days of illness are virtually identical to mild dengue, there follows a phase of profound, rapidly progressive, and potentially fatal illness, characterised by physical *shock* (collapse) and *haemorrhage* (bleeding). The skin is clammy, the limbs cold, the face exhibits blue mottling (cyanosis), the blood pressure is low (and often unrecordable), the pulse rapid and weak, and the liver enlarged. Bleeding is manifest in a variety of ways: from the nose (epistaxis), from the gums, in the urine (haematuria), in the vomit (haematemesis), in the stools (which are black and tarry), and in the skin (with

the appearance of blue/red spots, known as 'petechiae').
Death may occur in a matter of hours.

With regard to the treatment of dengue virus infections,
there are no orthodox antiviral agents available. Homoeopathic medicine, however, may be given along the following
lines:

(1) In the early stages of dengue, the following two
internal remedies should be given *in alternation (alternately)
every hour*:
    (a) *Aconite 30*
    (b) *Belladonna 30*
(2) Should the muscular or joint pains be excessive,
change to the following remedies, given *in alternation every
hour*:
    (a) *Eupatorium perfoliatum 6*
    (b) *Rhus toxicodendron 6*
(3) As an alternative to prescription (2), the following
two remedies may be given similarly *in alternation*:
    (a) *Bryonia 6*
    (b) *Rhus toxicodendron 6*
(4) Should the fever be diphasic ('saddleback'), in the
second phase the following two remedies are indicated,
given *in alternation every hour*:
    (a) *Gelsemium 6*
    (b) *Rhus toxicodendron 6*
(5) Where shock or haemorrhage (dengue haemorrhagic
fever) occur, intravenous and other supportive measures are
indicated, under expert medical supervision. Homoeopathically, remedies such as *Veratrum album* or *Carbo vegetabilis* may be helpful for the treatment of shock, whilst
others, such as *Crotalus horridus* or *Lachesis*, may reduce
the bleeding tendency.

> [where the available remedies differ in potency from
> those given above, in general they may be given with
> a similar frequency of repetition]

O'nyong-nyong
A benign dengue-like disease, occurring in epidemic form in Africa,
characterised by low fever, severe joint pains, an itchy skin rash, conjunc-

tivitis, inflammation of the palate, and enlargement of lymph nodes. Homoeopathically, Rhus toxicodendron may be helpful.

Lassa fever

This is yet another *viral haemorrhagic fever*, and is only of concern to those who visit or reside in West Africa. It is usually acquired by the consumption of food contaminated with infected rats' urine, and this is most likely to occur in those who choose to eat in primitive habitations.

The incubation period is generally 3–16 days. The disease is not of sudden onset, but develops gradually over the first 3–6 days. Its initial manifestations resemble *influenza*, with which it may be confused: feeling unwell, lack of appetite, sore throat, headache, muscular aches, and a gradual rise in temperature. There follows an abrupt deterioration in the patient's condition. Characteristically, white patches appear in the throat, which is extremely sore, rendering swallowing difficult (dysphagia). The lymph-glands in the neck enlarge, and swelling of the latter and the face occur. The temperature is now high, and the degree of prostration severe. There may be abdominal pain, diarrhoea, and vomiting. Symptoms resembling pneumonia may develop. Haemorrhage occurs, but is not severe: nose-bleed (epistaxis), coughing up blood (haemoptysis), or purple spots in the skin (purpura), which do not fade on pressure. Death occurs in 55% of untreated cases on days 7–14, from physical shock and toxicity.

Western physicians should be conversant with this serious disease, since it may occur in patients returning from rural West Africa, and it may be confused with more familiar illnesses, such as influenza, streptococcal tonsillitis, and glandular fever. Delay in treatment may have fatal consequences. Orthodox drug treatment is available, which reduces the mortality rate to 5%, but homoeopathy should not be forgotten, especially with regard to resistant cases, or in circumstances where conventional treatment is not to be found. The following two remedies, given either alone or in combination, should be considered:

(1) *Lachesis 6 4h*
(2) *Lassa fever nosode 30 4h*

Notes:

(i) For those nursing such patients, it is important to note that the virus may persist in the throat for 14 days, and in the urine for 35 days after the onset of the disease.

(ii) Two other diseases closely resemble Lassa fever in their symptomatic picture. Argentinian haemorrhagic fever occurs mainly in maize workers at harvest time, in the Buenos Aires, Cordoba, and Santa Fé provinces of Argentina. The infection is believed to be acquired by the inhalation of dried particles of infected field mouse urine, or the contact of abrasions with the same. The mortality rate is 10–20%. Bolivian haemorrhagic fever, for which the natural reservoir is the mouse, occurs in epidemic form in rural Bolivia, and has a mortality rate of 5–30%. Homoeopathic treatment might be along similar lines to those suggested for Lassa fever, using a nosode (*Lassa fever nosode*, or a specific nosode), plus other remedies, including those which are antihaemorrhagic, such as *Lachesis*.

Yellow fever

This viral disease, endemic in the tropical and subtropical regions of South and Central America and Africa, is transmitted by the bites of *Aedes* and jungle mosquitoes. Epidemics have even occurred far into the temperate zones during hot weather. The natural reservoir for infection is the monkey, and mosquitoes may transmit infection from monkey to man, or from man to man. See *Sections 3* and *14*, with regard to prevention.

The incubation period is 3–6 days. The disease is extremely variable in the severity of its manifestations, and many mild cases occur. In severe cases there is a *sudden* onset of fever, chills (shivering), muscle pains, bone pains, backache, severe headache, pain in the upper abdomen, vomiting, flushed face, coated tongue, and offensive breath. With regard to the evolution of the pulse, *Faget's sign* is characteristic: the pulse falls whilst the temperature remains constant, or the temperature rises whilst the pulse remains constant (a relative slowness of the pulse is also seen in typhoid, typhus, sandfly fever, and dengue). The maximum temperature is 40°C (104°F). After 3–4 days there may be some remission of the condition, and a fall in temperature. In mild cases this proceeds to recovery. In severe cases, however, after several hours or one day, the remission abates, and there follows a rapid deterioration in the disorder. The fever undergoes a secondary rise, producing a 'saddleback' (diphasic) curve on the temperature chart, rather like that of dengue (see above). Jaundice (yellow tint to the skin and the whites of the eyes), which subsequently intensifies, and haemorrhage generally become apparent by days 4–5. Nausea and vomiting are common, with the expulsion of the black vomit of altered blood in severe cases (an ominous sign). There may be purpura (purple spots on the skin, which do not fade on pressure), bleeding from the gums, nose-bleed (epistaxis), and black, tarry stools (melaena). The urine becomes scanty, dark, and thick, and will almost solidify on heating. In general, the patient is conscious and rational, but periods of confusion and delirium may occur. Coma precedes death, which occurs in approximately 50% of severe cases. In native populations in endemic areas the mortality rate is generally 7–10%. Most deaths occur during days 4–9, survival past day 10 indicating likely recovery. Relapses are rare, and permanent immunity is conferred.

Yellow fever must be differentiated from hepatitis, malaria, leptospirosis, and other forms of jaundice. Especially in mild cases, on clinical grounds alone, this may be difficult. The occurrence of fever in an unimmunized patient, during an outbreak of jaundice carrying a high mortality, is to be regarded with suspicion.

Apart from supportive measures, including the supply of fluid to oppose dehydration, orthodox medicine has no treatment for this disease. Homoeopathically, treatment with internal remedies along the following lines may be instituted:

(1) In all cases, the following may be given throughout, in conjunction with other indicated remedies:

Yellow fever nosode 30 6h

(2) In the early stages of the fever, give the following two remedies *in alternation (alternately) every hour*:
　(a) *Aconite 6*
　(b) *Belladonna 6*
(3) Should pain in the upper abdomen (epigastrium) occur, accompanied by severe back or bone pains, give the following two remedies *in alternation every hour*:

(a) *Bryonia 6*
(b) *Belladonna 6*

(4) After each episode of vomiting, give:

Ipecacuanha 6

(5) For sleeplessness and restlessness in a fully conscious patient, give:

Coffea cruda 6 ¼h

(6) If delirium occurs, give:

Hyoscyamus 6 ¼h

(7) If the fever persists, give:

Gelsemium 6 1h

(8) If dark haemorrhages occur, give the following two remedies *in alternation every hour*:
(a) *Crotalus horridus 6*
(b) *Arsenicum album 6*

(9) As an alternative to prescription (8), with the same indications, the following two remedies may be given, with similar frequency of alternation:
(a) *Lachesis 6*
(b) *Arsenicum album 6*

(10) After every bout of black vomit, give a single dose of:

Argentum nitricum 6

(11) If there are bright haemorrhages, purpuric spots of the skin, and marked jaundice, give:

Phosphorus 6 2h

(12) For suppression of urine, give the following two remedies *in alternation every hour*:
(a) *Apis mellifica 2x*
(b) *Opium 6*

(13) As a last resort, in serious cases, give:

Carbo vegetabilis 30 ¼h

(14) During convalescence, give:

Cinchona officinalis 6 6h

Acute hepatitis

A number of different viruses may produce acute inflammation of the liver, or *acute hepatitis*, as it is termed. From the traveller's point of view, the most important of these is the *Hepatitis A virus*. The transmission of *hepatitis A* is largely via food or drink contaminated with infected faecal material, and although it is of world-wide distribution, it is more common in situations where insanitary conditions prevail. The disease may present itself sporadically, or in an epidemic form. Another type of hepatitis, contracted in a similar manner, is *hepatitis E*, responsible for epidemics in Asia and North Africa. With regard to preventative measures, see *Sections 3* and *10*.

Hepatitis A is generally a self-limiting disease, with a low mortality rate (less than 0.2%), and one in which chronic (persistent) hepatitis does not occur as a sequel. Occasionally, however, the illness may be of a fulminating nature, with death occurring in a few days. The disease is more severe in the elderly.

The speed of onset of viral hepatitis of any type may be abrupt or insidious. The early symptoms include: feeling unwell (malaise), chilliness, chills (shivering), muscle pains, joint pains, sore throat, nasal discharge, severe lack of appetite, nausea, vomiting, and diarrhoea or constipation. The level of fever rarely exceeds 39.5°C (103.1°F), and the symptomatic picture of the initial illness may be mistaken for that of *influenza*. Mild upper abdominal pain, aggravated by jarring or movement, is often experienced on the right side. This may, though rarely, be severe. Tender enlargement of the liver is present in over 50% of cases, and enlargement of the spleen in 15%. Enlarged lymph-glands in the neck may be detected. Jaundice (yellow tint to the skin and eyes) may or may not occur. It may appear at the same time as the initial illness, or after 5–10 days after the onset of symptoms. The urine becomes dark. The acute illness usually lasts 2–3 weeks, followed by recovery. Full recovery occurs within 9 weeks of the onset of the disease in cases of hepatitis A.

Acute hepatitis with jaundice must be differentiated from other diseases, such as malaria, leptospirosis, and yellow fever. Apart from supportive measures, orthodox medicinal therapy is unavailable. Homoeopathically, in all cases of suspected viral hepatitis, irrespective of type (A, B, or E), give:

> *Phosphorus 6 6h*

To this may be added:

> *Hepatitis AB nosode 30 6h*

Sandfly fever (Phlebotomus fever)

This disease is transmitted by sandflies. See also *Sections 14 and 22*, with regard to the prevention of sandfly bites. It is found in Italy, the Adriatic coast of the former Yugoslavia, Greece, Crete, Cyprus, Malta, Egypt, Syria, Iraq, Iran, Israel, the Crimean coast, the Azov and Black Sea littoral, parts of the former USSR, and India. The incubation period is 3–4 days. Symptoms include: fever, headache, aversion to light, burning of the eyes, neck and back stiffness, back pain, joint and limb pains, nausea, vomiting, alteration or loss of taste, sore throat, profuse sweating, chilliness, chills (shivering), and initial constipation. *The exposed parts of the head and neck are very red, giving the appearance of severe sunburn.* In most cases, fever lasts 2–4 days (range: 1–9 days). The pulse is at first rapid, but then drops more rapidly than the temperature (relative slowness of the pulse is also seen in typhoid, dengue, yellow fever, and typhus). The pulse may remain slow during convalescence. Fatalities are unknown, but relapses may occur. Hot packs help to relieve the muscle pains. Homoeopathically, give the following two remedies *in alternation (alternately) every 1–2 hours*:

(a) *Belladonna 30*
(b) *Rhus toxicodendron 6*

Some other notable viral diseases

We shall now briefly consider a number of diseases which may be of importance to many. With regard to their homoeopathic treatment, the application of specific *nosodes*, prepared from diseased tissue containing the appropriate viruses, may be generally helpful. These would normally be given in a *30th potency 6–12h*, according to the severity of the condition. Additionally, other remedies, determinable by the symptomatic picture, may be utilised. Where possible, for those with some homoeopathic experience, remedies that might be applicable are given in parentheses.

(1) *Japanese B encephalitis*. See also *Sections 3* and *14*, with regard to prevention. One of the most important viral infections in India and South-East Asia, though of little concern to the urban traveller. Incubation period 6–8 days. Fever, followed by encephalitis (inflammation of the brain). Drowsiness, irritability, insomnia, and severe headache, progressing to paralysis, coma and death (20–65%). May be confused with cerebral malaria. [*Belladonna, Hyoscyamus, Opium*]

(2) *Poliomyelitis*. Infection is generally acquired by the ingestion of food or drink contaminated with faecal material. See also *Sections 3* and *10*, with regard to prevention. Fatalities may occur. Fever, nausea, vomiting, muscle weakness, headache, neck stiffness, and sore throat progress to a stage of paralysis. [*Lathyrus*]

(3) *Rift Valley fever*. South and East Africa, Egypt. Transmitted by mosquitoes (see *Section 14*). Incubation period: 3–7 days. Generally a self-limiting disease, lasting several days, with fever, headache, muscle and joint pains, and aversion to light (photophobia). Relapse and prolonged convalescence are rare. Only about 5% experience more severe symptoms, including jaundice and haemorrhage. [*Aconite, Belladonna, Rhus toxicodendron, Eupatorium perfoliatum*; with haemorrhages and jaundice: *Crotalus horridus, Lachesis*]

(4) *Ross River fever*. An epidemic form of polyarthritis (inflammation of joints), spread by mosquitoes. See also *Section 14*, with regard to the prevention of mosquito bites.

This disease occurs not only in the Ross River area of Australia, but also in the Cook and Samoan Islands, Fiji, the Solomon and other islands of Melanesia. Almost all cases occur between December and June. The onset of the disease is marked by headache, mild nasal catarrh, and tenderness of the palms and soles. Fever is absent or mild, and, if present, does not exceed 38° C (100.4° F). The two important features are arthritis, and a skin rash. In 50% of cases, joint symptoms occur 1–15 days before the rash is apparent. In the remainder, the rash precedes the arthritis by 2–10 days. The rash is slightly raised (maculopapular), and usually begins on the cheeks and forehead, spreading to the trunk. It may be itchy, and, in some cases, vesicles (small fluid-filled blisters) appear. The arthritis mainly involves the small joints of the fingers and hands, but the wrists and ankles may also be affected. There is pain, and swelling may occur in some cases. 20% of cases exhibit tender enlargement of the lymph-glands. The joint symptoms may persist for 3–12 weeks. [*Rhus toxicodendron, Bryonia*]

(5) *Colorado tick fever.* A disease limited to the western USA, and transmitted by ticks, principally between March and August. See *Section 14* with regard to prevention. Incubation period: 1–19 days. The onset is abrupt, with high fever (up to 40.6° C/105° F), severe muscle pains, chills (shivering), headache, vomiting, prostration, and sometimes a faint rash becomes visible. Typically, the fever lasts for 3 days, followed by a remission for 1–3 days, followed by a full relapse for 2–4 days. Occasionally, three bouts of fever may occur. Whilst complications may arise (meningitis, encephalitis, haemorrhage), the disease is usually benign and self-limiting (although residual weakness may be present for some time after). It must be differentiated from Rocky Mountain spotted fever, and influenza. [*Rhus toxicodendron, Eupatorium perfoliatum, Kali phosphoricum*]

(6) *European tick-borne encephalitis.* Symptoms similar to those of Japanese B encephalitis (see above). See also *Sections 3* and *14*.

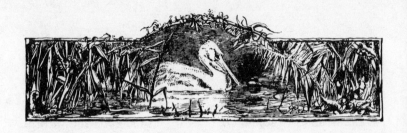

Section 25

THE TYPHUS FAMILY

Rickettsiae, a group of microorganisms which resemble bacteria in form, are, however, obligatory intracellular parasites; rather like viruses, they are confined within the bounds of the host cell. They are generally transmitted to man by various arthropods, and the principal diseases produced are known generically as *typhus*. With regard to preventative measures, see *Sections 3, 14, and 16*.

Epidemic louse-borne typhus

This disease, associated with famine, deprivation, overcrowding, and insanitary conditions, is disseminated by the human body louse. In the present era, it is largely found in South America, Africa, and Asia. It is of little concern to those who stay in respectable accommodation. The incubation period is 10–14 days. There is an initial (prodromal) phase of headache, backache, joint pains, and chest pains. There abruptly follow high fever, chills (shivering), and severe and intractable headache; later there may be delirium. The eyes are inflamed, the face flushed, and the spleen is often enlarged. Clinical identification of the disease rests mainly on the characteristic skin rash that appears. Typically this arises between days 3–7, first in the arm-pits and on the flanks, progressing to the chest and back, being most marked on the latter. Later, this spreads to the extremities, but the palms and soles are seldom affected, and the face remains clear. Initially it is composed of slightly raised, dusky rose spots, which blanch on pressure, and may become confluent. Later, they may become purpuric (purple and haemorrhagic, not blanching on pressure), and, during convalescence, they become brownish, and gradually fade. With the onset of the rash, the patient's condition worsens, and foulness of the mouth, cough, and constipation may be present. In cases of spontaneous improvement, this generally occurs between days 13–16, with a fall in temperature, and return to normality. Complications include: bronchitis, pneumonia, kidney failure (uraemia), inflammation of the heart (myocarditis), middle ear infection (otitis media), and gangrene of the toes, fingers, or of the skin overlying the lowest part of the back (sacrum). The mortality rate is partially dependent upon age, being low in children under 10, 10% at ages 10–30, and 60% in those over 50. Even after recovery from the initial attack, dormant rickettsiae may become reactivated, sometimes years later, to produce a usually milder form of the disease (*Brill's disease*), associated with a low mortality.

Endemic flea-borne typhus (Murine typhus)
This disease, of world-wide distribution throughout areas of warmer climate, is transmitted to humans by the bite of the rat flea. This is altogether a milder disease than primary louse-borne typhus, and more closely resembles *Brill's disease* (see above). The onset is more gradual, the duration shorter (6–13 days), and the intensity of symptoms less than that described above for its louse-borne relative. Pneumonia, gangrene, and fatality are rare, and any deaths are usually confined to the elderly.

Scrub typhus (Tsutsugamushi disease/Mite typhus)
This disease is found widely in East and South Asia, the islands of the western Pacific, and Australia. It is transmitted by larval mites, known as *chiggers* (not to be confused with 'jiggers', which are parasitic fleas, and nothing to do with typhus). Those walking through vegetation, especially long grass, become victims, and since there is seldom any marked

itch, they are usually unaware of exposure to possible infection. The incubation period is 7–18 days. Characteristically, in 50–80% of cases, a black *eschar*, an ulcer 2–4mm across, may be located at the site of the mite attachment. Often this will be in the region of the genitalia or arm-pits, but may be elsewhere. Occasionally, several eschars may be present. The general symptoms of the initial illness include: severe headache, chilliness, and fever. During the first week there is a progressive increase in temperature, reaching 40–40.5°C (104–105°F), whilst the pulse remains relatively slow, usually not exceeding 100 beats/minute (slowness of the pulse is also seen in typhoid, dengue, yellow fever, and sandfly fever). The lymph-glands draining the area of the original bite become enlarged and tender. Other lymph-glands elsewhere may also increase in size, though less markedly, and the spleen may enlarge. Between days 5–10, a characteristic flat red rash appears on the trunk, which may extend to the limbs. The rash is of brief duration, seldom persisting for more than several days, though occasionally for a week. During the second week the temperature remains high, but the pulse increases. There may be conjunctivitis (red eyes), deafness, headache, apathy, and confusion. In severe cases there may be delirium, and twitching of the muscles. Cough is common, and in more than 50% of cases, this is associated with pneumonia. Inflammation of the heart (myocarditis), and heart failure may occur. The mortality rate may be in the range of 10–60%. In cases of spontaneous recovery, the fever falls at the end of the second week, or the beginning of the third. A prolonged convalescent period is usual, and there may be residual deafness, and psychological abnormalities.

Scrub typhus must be differentiated from malaria, leptospirosis, dengue, and typhoid.

Tick typhus (Spotted fever)

Fièvre boutonneuse, *Kenya tick typhus*, *South African tick fever*, and *Indian tick typhus* are all caused by essentially the same species of rickettsia, and are all transmitted by the bite of a tick. The geographical areas of risk are the Mediterranean, Africa, and India. These diseases are generally mild in nature, and are characterised by the presence of an eschar (see above), painful enlargement of the regional lymph-glands, a slightly raised rash focussed on the trunk (sometimes with small haemorrhages, termed 'petechiae'), appearing around day 5, and signs of brain disturbance, including slowness of response, stupor, or confusion. The eyes and face may be red, and headache and muscular pains may be bothersome. The mortality rate, however, is negligible, and spontaneous resolution occurs within a few weeks. *Siberian tick typhus* (Siberia and Mongolia), and *North Queensland tick typhus* (North and South Queensland, Australia) are similar in character and intensity.

In contrast, *Rocky Mountain spotted fever* is a variety of tick typhus that may be associated with severe symptoms and consequences. Whilst mild cases do occur, the mortality rate in the untreated may be as high as 70% in the elderly, or as low as 20% in children. Infection is transmitted by the wood tick in the western USA, and by the dog tick in the eastern USA. The disease has also been reported in the southern USA, Canada (British Columbia, Alberta, Saskatchewan), Mexico, Panama, Brazil, and Colombia. Most cases occur in late spring or summer. The incubation period is 3–14 days. Except in Brazil, an eschar (see above) is not found. Initial influenza-like symptoms give way to chills (shivering), high fever, severe headache, severe muscular and joint pains, great restlessness, and prostration. There may be delirium, or even coma. A characteristic flat red rash appears between days 2–6 of the fever, beginning on the wrists and ankles, then spreading centrally to the arms, legs, and trunk. The rash becomes slightly raised, and then petechiae appear. Complications include: jaundice, gangrene, kidney failure, and heart failure. Where spontaneous resolution occurs, this is generally around the end of the second week. Improvement is then rapid, and convalescence short. The rash of Rocky Mountain spotted fever may be confused with that of typhoid, meningococcal infection, or measles.

Special tests may be helpful with regard to establishing a diagnosis with regard to any form of typhus.

Treatment of the typhus group

Orthodox treatment is available. With regard to homoeopathic therapy, the following guide-lines may be given:

(1) Specific *nosodes* (prepared from appropriate diseased tissue), given in the *30th potency 6–12h, according to severity*, may be given throughout, in conjunction with other indicated remedies.

(2) In mild cases, with muscular or joint pains, and great restlessness:

Rhus toxicodendron 6 1h

(3) In severe cases, with much drowsiness or delirium:

Baptisia 30 1h

(4) In severe cases, with much anxiety, thirst for sips, chilliness despite a high temperature:

Arsenicum album 6 1h

(5) Where pneumonia is suspected, add:

Phosphorus 6 1h

(6) Where there is significant enlargement of the regional lymph-glands:

Mercurius solubilis 6 2h

Trench fever

A self-limiting louse-borne rickettsial disease, endemic in Central America. Abrupt onset. Fever lasts 3–5 days. Weakness, severe pain behind the eyes, and in the back and legs. Transient rash may appear. Sometimes enlargement of spleen and lymph nodes. Relapses occur. Rhus toxicodendron may be indicated.

Q fever

A rickettsial infection often acquired by drinking unpasteurised milk, and sometimes by the inhalation of contaminated dust originating from infected animals (cattle, sheep, goats). World-wide distribution. Sore throat, red eyes, and cough. Illness usually resolves in 1–3 weeks, but may lie dormant, only to reappear later in the form of various serious heart and brain disorders. A specific homoeopathic nosode might be considered.

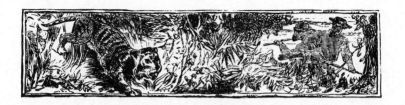

SOME IMPORTANT PARASITES

In this section are considered three important parasitic diseases: *kala azar*, *Chagas' disease*, and *African sleeping sickness*.

Kala azar (Visceral leishmaniasis)
Before proceeding with this topic, you should familiarise yourself with that part of *Section 22* devoted to *cutaneous and mucocutaneous leishmaniasis*. Kala azar, caused by various subspecies of the protozoan parasite *Leishmania donovani*, is similarly transmitted by the bites of sandflies; and occasionally, via blood transfusion. It is found in the Mediterranean area (including North Africa), the Middle East, central Asia, China, parts of Central and South America, India, and tropical Africa. Whilst the disease is rare in ordinary travellers, even those who visit such places as southern Spain, the South of France, North Africa, and mainland Greece (especially Athens and Piraeus) may succumb. In the Mediterranean region and South America, where the natural animal reservoirs are the dog and the fox, kala azar is mainly a disease of infants and young children. In India there appears to be no animal reservoir, except man himself.

In the Sudan, various rodents harbour the disease. The recognition of this illness is of paramount importance, since, without appropriate treatment, death is usually the outcome within 3–24 months. The dominant cause of death is secondary infection, particularly of the lungs or gut; pneumonia, tuberculosis, and amoebic or bacillary dysentery are all common. The disease may present in the form of fever, wasting, and diarrhoea. In non-endemic countries, the diagnosis may be easily missed in cases with a long incubation period (see below). The infection may have been acquired many months (or even years) before, whilst on a trip to an endemic zone. Moreover, the disease may simulate other diseases, more commonly prevalent in non-endemic areas, such as leukaemia or cancer of the lymphatic system, thus throwing the physician off the scent. Special tests are always helpful.

Rarely, and mainly in cases from the Sudan, a small nodule, or what appears to be an oriental sore (see *Section 22*) becomes apparent at the site of the sandfly bite, this preceding the onset of general symptoms by 4–6 months. Occasionally, the Mediterranean variety of *Leishmania donovani* infection presents similarly, but the disease remains locally in the skin, and does not progress to disseminated infection; this, presumably, as a result of a high immune status. Also in the Sudan, the disease may present with lesions resembling espundia (see *Section 22*), with erosions of the mouth or nose, and with or without signs of more generalised kala azar. In most cases, initial skin signs will be absent.

The incubation period can be anything from 10 days to 2 years, with a few exceptional cases occurring up to 9 years after infection. The disease may be abrupt or insidious in onset. In travellers and expatriate residents, it usually begins suddenly, with a high fever, chills (shivering), and profuse sweating. Characteristically, in 20% of patients, the temperature shows a double rise in 24 hours, resembling that of malignant malaria. The fever increases in the early afternoon, diminishes towards the evening, and rises again, usually before midnight. The initial fever may last 2–6 weeks, and sometimes longer. Subsequently, waves of fever separated by periods of normal temperature may resemble the pattern seen in brucellosis (see *Section 23*). Paradoxically, the patient feels reasonably well and will go about the day's activities, often quite unaware of the febrile state. The appetite is good, the tongue clean, and the mind clear and active. This is quite different from the symptomatic picture seen in malaria or typhoid. The spleen enlarges, often considerably, although an increase in size, in some cases, is not discernible until the fifth month of illness. Some enlargement of the liver may also occur. As the disease progresses, a characteristic greyish pigmentation appears in the skin, usually most noticeable on the forehead, the central line of the abdomen, the hands, and the nails (hence, *kala azar* = black fever). Anaemia is also manifest.

In the indigenous populace of endemic areas the onset of the disease is often more insidious. The fever is often low, and subsequently may exhibit great variation in pattern. Commonly, the dominant complaint, especially in children, is pain under the ribs on the left side, and swelling of the abdomen, both due to enlargement of the spleen. The skin becomes rough and develops the characteristic greyish pigmentation, the hair becomes brittle and sparse, the legs may become swollen and bruised (purpura), and jaundice may be present. Cough is not an uncommon symptom, and, in some cases, may be associated with tuberculosis of the lungs.

Whenever a person presents with loss of weight, anaemia, fever, and enlargement of the spleen, with a history of a visit to, or residency within, an endemic area, within 9 years of onset of the disorder, the possibility of kala azar as a diagnosis should be strongly considered.

With regard to therapy, orthodox drug treatment is available, but some infections may be resistant to treatment, and relapses may occur. Homoeopathically, many different remedies might be indicated, according to individual symptoms, but the following more specific comments may be made:

(1) In all cases, in conjunction with other remedies, the following may be given:

Kala azar nosode 30 once weekly

(2) In cases of Mediterranean infantile kala azar, the following may be found helpful:

Arsenicum album 6 6h

(3) Additionally, either of the following two spleen remedies may be given:

(a) *Ceanothus americanus 12h*

(b) *Quercus glandium spiritus 10 drops 6h*

[reduce the dose of (b) for children]

Chagas' disease (American trypanosomiasis)

This essentially rural disease, caused by the protozoan parasite *Trypanosoma cruzi*, is entirely limited in its distribution to the Americas. It is found extensively throughout non-urban Central and South America, and Mexico. Occasional cases have been reported in the USA (Texas). It is estimated that some 12 million people are infected with this disease, of which about 60,000 die annually, usually from heart disease, of which it is the most significant cause in South America.

The disease is transmitted by *kissing bugs*, so called because of their predilection for biting the cheek. They are also termed *assassin bugs*, presumably because they attack stealthily at night, whilst the victim is asleep. Kissing bugs, which are about 1–4cm (½-1½in) in length, are largely found in poor dwellings, such as huts and hovels. The average traveller, who stays in respectable accommodation, should have little fear of infection. The disease may also be transmitted congenitally and by blood transfusion.

The microparasite, contained within the faeces of the bug, either enters through the bite wound, or through the conjunctiva of the eye. In most cases, infection remains within the body, causes no immediate symptoms, and lies dormant for many years (*latent phase*). In some cases, however, an initial *acute phase* is evident. *Acute Chagas' disease*, as it is termed, is mainly seen in children. The earliest signs are at the point of inoculation. If in the skin, a tender swelling, known as a *chagoma*, appears, resembling a blind boil (furuncle), which persists for many months. If in the eye, *Romaña's sign* is observed: unilateral severe swelling of upper and lower eyelids, conjunctivitis, and enlargement of the lymph-glands under the jaw on the same side. After 7–

14 days, more general symptoms arise. There is an abrupt onset of fever, which may be high, and persist for many weeks. Sometimes the temperature chart shows a double spike in 24 hours (see above, under *kala azar*). The patient feels unwell, and generalised enlargement of the lymph-nodes occurs. Moderate enlargement of the spleen and liver are found. The pulse rate remains rapid, even as the temperature falls. Inflammation of the testicle may be present. In severe forms of the disease, inflammation of the heart or brain often results in death, this occurring in up to 10% of acute cases. The majority of patients recover spontaneously in 4–8 weeks, but then enter the *latent phase*.

The *latent phase*, which may last 10–30 years, is entered either directly after inoculation with the parasite (the majority of cases), or after surviving the acute illness (especially children). As has been stated, the parasite lies dormant, and no symptoms are produced.

The *chronic phase*, which follows the latent phase, generally arises between the ages of 20–30. It is characterised by severe heart disorders, often leading to death in 5–6 years, and enlargement of the large gut and oesophagus, leading to constipation, difficulty in swallowing, and regurgitation of food.

Special tests are available to confirm the diagnosis. Orthodox drug treatment is available, but is unsatisfactory. It is either excessively toxic, or ineffective. Homoeopathically, the following suggestions may be made:

(1) In acute cases, in addition to other indicated remedies, consider:

Chagas' nosode 30 6h

(2) In latent and chronic cases, in addition to other indicated remedies, consider long-term administration of:

Chagas' nosode 30–200 once every 1–4 weeks

(3) In acute cases, with Romaña's sign:

Kali carbonicum 6 6h

(4) In acute cases, with chagoma:

Ledum 6 6h

(5) Various supportive remedies may be required in chronic cases, eg: *Phosphorus* for regurgitation, *Alumina* for constipation, *Crataegus ø* for heart disease.

African sleeping sickness (African trypanosomiasis)

Untreated, most people who acquire this serious disease will die. Sleeping sickness, of which there are two varieties, is caused by the protozoan parasite *Trypanosoma brucei gambiense* in West Africa, and by *Trypanosoma brucei rhodesiense* in East Africa. The vectors of both types of disease are various species of *tsetse fly*. In East Africa, the tsetse flies are to be found in woodland and bush, whereas their West African cousins are found near rivers and streams. The main reservoirs of infection are man in West Africa, and wild game in East Africa.

The principal areas of risk to the traveller to East or West Africa, are, therefore, rivers and streams in the latter, and game reserves in the former. Urban areas are essentially safe. The tsetse fly, about the size of a common housefly, bites in the day, and is particularly attracted to moving vehicles, and the colour dark blue. All safari vehicles should have their windows tightly closed, and the passenger compartment should be regularly sprayed with *pyrethrum*. Those on foot or on horseback are less likely to be bitten. Insect repellents may be partially effective, but great reliance should not be put upon them. Clothing should cover as much of the body as possible.

The East African infection, which exhibits three stages, is significantly more virulent than that of West Africa, and death may occur within weeks to one year. In contrast, the West African disease is more insidious: the first stage, involving the skin and regional lymph-glands, is absent; the second stage, with general symptoms, moderate or absent; the third stage, involving the brain, mild in onset, with death occurring in 2–3 years.

The first stage: local reaction. About 2 days after a tsetse bite, a dusky red swelling appears at the site of the latter, resembling a blind boil, but relatively painless. This lesion, hot to the touch, may be 2–5cm in diameter, and remains present for 2–4 weeks. Accompanying this *trypanosomal chancre*, which is more common in Caucasians than Africans, there is enlargement of the regional lymph-glands.

The second stage: general invasion. 5–21 days after the infecting bite, general symptoms make their appearance. Irregular waves of fever, severe headache, and aches and pains occur, interspersed with symptomless periods of up to 14 days. Rapidity of the pulse persists during these intermissions. Enlargement of the spleen and liver may be manifest, and swelling around the eyes, and of the hands and feet may be present. Itchy rashes often appear. Enlarged and painless lymph-glands are present in 75% of patients, but in the East African disease only those at the back of the neck are so affected (Winterbottom's sign). An excessive feeling of pain in response to touch or pressure (Kerandel's sign) is occasionally detected, this response being particularly apparent in the shins. Increasing weight loss, anaemia, and weakness develop. Inflammation of the heart may arise, with death occurring before the third stage is entered.

The third stage: brain disease. In the East African disease, this stage generally arises within a few weeks or months of initial infection, whereas, in the West African variety, it occurs insidiously between 6 months and several years after this event. Initial signs include: mood swings, personality change, argumentative or difficult behaviour, neglect of personal appearance, and apathy. Later: difficulty in walking, speaking, and feeding, tremors, and fits. The somnolence that gives the name to the disease is late in appearance. Emaciated, the patient dies in coma, or from secondary infection.

Sleeping sickness, which may be confirmed by means of special tests, may be mistaken for other diseases such as malaria, influenza, glandular fever, and various psychiatric disorders. Orthodox drug therapy is available, and is highly effective in many cases, provided that deterioration of the nervous system is not advanced. Homoeopathically, the following may be indicated:

(1) A specific *nosode* (made from diseased tissue) may

303

be used throughout, in addition to other indicated remedies. According to the type of disease, use either *East African sleeping sickness nosode*, or *West African sleeping sickness nosode*:

- (a) East African type, stages 1 and 2: *30th potency 6–12h.*
- (b) East African type, stage 3; West African type, stages 2 and 3: *30–200th potency once weekly*.

(2) Emaciation, great weakness, swellings, depression:

Arsenicum album 6–30 6h

[well-suited to many cases]

(3) Weakness with Kerandel's sign (hypersensitivity to touch/pressure):

Cinchona officinalis 6–30 6h

(4) Slowness of mind, answers slowly, stammering, swellings, drowsiness:

Plumbum metallicum 6 6h

(5) Lethargy, drowsiness, but awakes with great fear or anxiety:

Opium 30 6h

Other homoeopathic remedies in sleeping sickness

Antimonium tartaricum, Calcarea phosphorica, Ferrum metallicum, Kali carbonicum, Manganum, Natrum muriaticum, Nux moschata, Phosphorus.

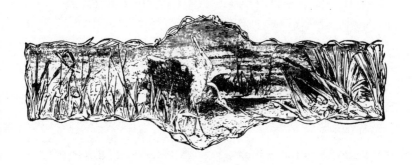

Section 27

ASSORTED WORMS

In this, the final major section of the manual, a variety of important parasitic worm infestations will be considered. However, before we proceed with a consideration of each individually, it is pertinent to make some general comments with regard to therapy.

It is essential to realise that, especially in the tropics, worm infections are extremely common, that most are light, barely, if at all, affecting the health of the host, and that, even with successful treatment, reinfection is frequent in those who are resident. Hence, treatment should be restricted to those in whom the health has been impaired, and, of the remainder, to only those in whom reinfection is unlikely, viz. some residents, and most travellers.

With regard to actual therapy, this may be achieved in two cardinal ways. Firstly, the worms may be poisoned, or expelled by orthodox drugs or botanic medicines. Secondly, homoeopathic remedies may be administered, which, by acting on the host rather than the worm, render the tissues less receptive to such infection.

In some instances, homoeopathy by itself will totally rid the host of the parasitic worm. This is frequently the case in most threadworm infections. However, in many situations, the effect is a lesser one. There may be both a laudable improvement in health, as witnessed by a reduction of symptoms, and a decrease in the number of worms; but, whilst the patient enters into a new and happier relationship with the invader, total elimination may not be possible by homoeopathic means. For those who might suffer reinfection, particularly the indigenous population of an area who are unable to reform matters such as hygiene, this may be a satisfactory result. For others, it may be less than satisfactory. Indeed, where it is the intention of the practitioner to rid the person totally of infestation, it may be necessary to elicit the assistance of orthodox or botanic medicines, in order to poison or purge. It should be remembered, however, that, whilst homoeopathic remedies are essentially non-toxic to the host, the same cannot always be said for orthodox or botanic medicines. Some price, be it small or large, must be paid for their use.

It may be assumed, therefore, that the treatment of parasitic worms is a matter of selective judgement, according to the circumstances of the patient, and the availability of medicines. Homoeopathic and orthodox or botanic medicines may be used sequentially, in combination, or individually, in order to secure the desired result, as determined by sensible intention and therapeutic knowledge. With regard to the diseases described below, we shall, however, largely restrict ourselves to a consideration of the use of homoeopathic remedies, or other non-toxic measures. In addition to these, the value of homoeopathic *constitutional* treatment, prescribed by a professional homoeopathist (on the basis of the general characteristics of the patient), should be emphasised.

Threadworms (Pinworms/Enterobiasis)
These are slender, white, parasitic roundworms (*Enterobius vermicularis*), up to 1cm (½in) long, of world-wide distribution, and commoner in children. These worms inhabit the gut, the female emerging from the anus at night, in order to lay her eggs. This gives rise to the dominant symptom of itching around the anus. General symptoms may arise, including: loss of appetite and weight, bed-wetting, psychological insta-

bility, restlessness, and irritability. Infection is acquired through poor hygiene (usually, contaminated fingers to mouth). Homoeopathically, consider:

(1) In general:

Cina 30–200 12h

(2) Should this fail, administer the following remedies sequentially:
    (a) *Lycopodium 30 6h for 2 days,* followed by
    (b) *Veratrum album 30 6h for 4 days,* followed by
    (c) *Ipecacuanha 6 6h for 4 days*

Ascariasis (Long roundworms)

It is estimated that over 600 million people are infected with *Ascaris lumbricoides*, the most common parasitic roundworm in man. It is found in Africa, the Americas, Europe, and Asia. It is highly prevalent in China, South-East Asia, the central Asian republics of the former USSR, Latin America, and Africa. In some of these areas, as many as 95% of the population may be infected.

These are the largest of the intestinal roundworms, white to pink in colour, achieving a length of up to 35cm (14in). Human infection is acquired by the ingestion of eggs contained within soil, which may remain infective for up to 10 years after deposition via the faeces of the host. Vegetables are a common vector. Most infections are without symptoms, but the passage of worms in the faeces, or their appearance in vomit or the nostrils will signify their presence. Severe itching around the anus may be occur in some cases. Heavy infections, however, where 100 or more worms are present, may result in serious complications.

In children there may be nausea, vomiting, diarrhoea, and malnutrition. The latter may manifest as the protein-deficiency state known as *kwashiorkor*, vitamin A deficiency, leading to night blindness (which rapidly improves within days of reduction or elimination of the worm population), or vitamin C deficiency. Convulsions and epilepsy are seen occasionally. Obstruction of the gut by a ball of worms gives rise to severe abdominal pain and distention, vomiting and fever. Invasion of the biliary system, common in India, may lead to jaundice, and liver abscess. Round-worms and liver flukes (see below) are a frequent cause of acute inflammation of the pancreas in Hong Kong. The passage of worms through the lungs may cause fever, wheezing, breathlessness, cough, pain under the breast-bone, and nettle-rash (urticaria/hives), with spontaneous improvement in 5–10 days.

Surgery may be required in cases of obstruction to the gut or biliary system. Homoeopathic treatment includes:

(1) In general, in cases without serious complications, give the following for several weeks:

Viola odorata 6 6h

(2) Where the above fails:

Teucrium marum 6 6h

(3) In cases with lung symptoms:

Stannum metallicum 30 24h

Kwashiorkor and marasmus

Kwashiorkor, essentially due to insufficient protein, is a form of malnutrition commonly seen in children during times of famine. It is characterised by: swollen face, hands, and feet, thin upper arms, retardation of growth, wasting of muscles, sores and peeling of the skin, and loss of pigmentation of skin and hair. Marasmus, on the other hand, is due to not eating enough food generally, but especially energy foods (carbohydrates and fats). The child is small, very thin, wasted, very underweight, always hungry, and has a pot-belly. The upper arm test is a useful indicator of malnutrition in the less obvious early stages. If, after 1 year of age, the maximum circumference of the upper arm is less than 13cm, then the child is suffering from malnutrition; less than 12cm denotes severe malnutrition.

Trichuriasis (Whipworms)

This roundworm infection of the gut, of world-wide distribution, is more prevalent in warm and humid climates. It is acquired in a similar manner to Ascariasis (see above), and, indeed, the two may coexist in the same person. The whipworm, *Trichuris trichiura*, attains a length of up to 5cm (2in). The majority of whipworm infections are devoid of symptoms, but heavy infections in children, with up to 1000 worms, may cause severe symptoms. These include: profuse diarrhoea with blood and mucus (but no fever), abdominal pain, pain in the rectum (back passage), which may prolapse (project through the anus), wasting, and anaemia.

Homoeopathic therapy for cases with few symptoms may be given as listed above for *Ascariasis* (prescription 1 or 2). For cases with severe symptoms, including prolapse:

> *Podophyllum 6 6h*

Some tapeworms (flat, segmented worms)

Infection with *Taenia saginata*, the beef tapeworm, is particularly common in Africa, South America, and the Middle East. This ribbon-like worm, which may grow to a length of 20 metres (over 20yds) within the intestine, is acquired by eating *raw or undercooked* infected beef. Those who eat *steak a la tartare* in fashionable restaurants in Europe do so with some risk. Serious symptoms are rare, but some experience recurrent abdominal pain, and others suffer the discomfort of a worm segment wriggling through the anus. Often, the only finding is the odd worm segment in the faeces.

The dwarf tapeworm, *Hymenolepis nana*, in contrast, is no longer than 40mm (1½in). It is not uncommon in Latin America, India, the Mediterranean area, Egypt, and Sudan. It is acquired by eating food contaminated with infected mouse droppings. As with the beef tapeworm, it is confined to the intestine, and seldom causes symptoms. However, heavy infections in children may lead to abdominal pain, itching of the anus, diarrhoea, and vomiting.

Diphyllobothrium latum, the fish tapeworm, another intestinal parasite, may grow up to 10 metres (over 10yds) in length. Infection is acquired by eating *raw, undercooked, or pickled* fish, and is most prevalent in Manchuria, Japan (beware of *sushi*), South–East Asia, Europe, North America, and central Africa. Virtually all infections are without symptoms, but *vitamin B12* deficiency may arise in some cases.

A simple, extremely safe, and reasonably natural method

of expelling tapeworms, using fresh pumpkin seeds (*Cucurbita pepo* or *Cucurbita maxima*), is as follows:

(1) The patient must fast (or eat very little) for 12–16 hours.

(2) 60g (2oz) of fresh pumpkin seeds are scalded with boiling water. The outer skins are removed, and the green inner pulp (approximately 30g/1oz) retained. This pulp is ground to a paste with a little milk, and administered to the patient by mouth, after the fast.

(3) 2 hours later, a castor oil (*Oleum Ricini*) purge is given by mouth. This should be given in milk or fruit juice: *10–20ml of castor oil for adults, or 5–10ml for children 5–12 years of age*.

(4) The tapeworm is generally expelled 2–3 hours later.

Larval worm infections
Though less common an infective parasite than the beef tapeworm, the pork tapeworm, *Taenia solium*, differs in that it may give rise to serious disease. Simple infection of the intestine by the consumption of *raw or undercooked* pork is relatively innocuous, as with the beef or fish tapeworm, and it may, indeed, be expelled with the method given above. However, under certain circumstances, with or without the presence of an intestinal adult, the larval (immature) form of the worm is capable of invading the tissues of the body (*Cysticercosis*). This phenomenon may originate in a number of ways, all of which involve the passage of tapeworm eggs to the stomach (where their outer covering dissolves), and their subsequent penetration of the upper small intestine (duodenum). The eggs may be ingested in contaminated food, or acquired by oro-anal contact during heterosexual or homosexual intimacy. Alternatively, one's own eggs may be transferred by dirty fingers from anus to mouth. The larval worms give rise to cysts in muscles, and in the tissue immediately beneath the skin. Worse still, they may produce cysts within the brain. There is often a considerable delay between the time of infection and the onset of symptoms, from 5 months to 30 years. Serious symptoms include: persistent headache, and epilepsy. Many mild cases occur with virtually no symptoms.

Trichinosis, caused by the small roundworm, *Trichinella spiralis*, and its larval form, is of world-wide distribution. It is acquired by eating *raw or undercooked* bear meat (Thailand), pork (Hong Kong and elsewhere), bush pig or warthog (Africa), and walrus (Arctic). Upon consumption of infected meat, the gastric juices release larval worms from the cysts that contain them. These rapidly mature and mate to produce worms up to 3mm (⅛in) in length, the females of which then burrow into the lining of the small intestine, and produce new larvae, which proceed to invade the tissues of the body. These larvae give rise to inflammation, and, in the case of muscular tissue, cyst formation follows. Mild infections may display few or no symptoms. Heavy infections, on the other hand, will produce a severe reaction. Following ingestion of the parasite, there is an incubation period of ½-28 days. Initial symptoms, which last from 1–7 days, include: feeling unwell, abdominal cramps, and diarrhoea; less commonly, nausea, vomiting, and constipation. The second stage, which lasts from about day 7 to day 40 is associated with: painful and tender muscles (worse for movement), swelling around the eyes, conjunctivitis, cough, various haemorrhages (including splinter-like bleeds under the nails), and rashes. Severe neurological disorders may sometimes occur, such as paralysis and coma. Irregularity of the pulse, pneumonia, and inflammation of the kidneys are not unknown. Sudden death may occur. Recovery usually begins somewhere between day 35 and day 90, but muscle pains and malaise (feeling unwell) may be persistent for several months. Without treatment, the larval cysts remain viable for many years.

Hydatidosis, caused by the larval form of the canine tapeworm, *Echinococcus granulosus*, occurs mainly in areas where dogs are involved in the control of herds of grazing animals, especially sheep. The disease is prevalent in South America, the Middle East, central Asia, East Africa (especially the Turkana district of northern Kenya), and the Mediterranean littoral. It is also found in other areas of Europe, North America, Australasia, and India. The accidental ingestion of dog faeces containing eggs results in the disease. Invading the tissues, the larvae produce cysts, which may reach some considerable size. The majority of cysts occur in the liver, but may not be noticed until a period of 10–20 years has elapsed. Such cysts may produce nausea, vomiting, pain in the right side of the upper abdomen, and jaundice. In about 10% of cases, cysts occur in the lungs. Other sites include the brain, bones, spleen, kidneys, and muscles. With sufficient growth, symptoms ascribable to each structure will eventually occur.

Orthodox treatment of larval worm infection includes both drugs and surgery. Homoeopathically, the following may assist in securing a cure:

(1) In all types, to retard or reduce cysts:

Silicea 6 6h

(2) For the muscle pains of trichinosis, add:

Bryonia 30 6h

(3) For liver cysts in hydatidosis, add either of the following:
    (a) *Lycopodium 6 6h*
    (b) *Chelidonium majus 6 6h*

Oriental liver flukes (flatworms)

Infection is acquired by eating *raw* fish. *Opisthorchiasis*, caused by the liver fluke *Opisthorchis viverrini*, is highly prevalent in northern Thailand, where a principal source of infection is the dish known as *Koi-pla*. The other major liver fluke of South-East Asia, especially common in Hong Kong, is *Clonorchis sinensis*, causing the disease *clonorchiasis*. Both diseases are similar, often producing an enlarged and tender liver (which feels hot to the patient), intermittent fever, and jaundice. Abscess or cancer of the liver, and acute inflammation of the pancreas may also feature in the illness.

In addition to other measures, the following homoeopathic remedies may be helpful:

(1) Where there is a sensation of heat in the liver, either of these two remedies should be considered:
    (a) *Aloe 6 6h*
    (b) *Kali carbonicum 6 6h*

(2) Otherwise, or where the above fail, consider either of the following:
- (a) *Chelidonium majus 6 6h*
- (b) *Lycopodium 6 6h*

Human hookworm disease (Ancylostomiasis)

This disease is found in all tropical and subtropical areas of the World, including the southern USA, and western Australia. The eggs of the hookworm, which are deposited in soil via the faeces, hatch in warm and moist conditions to produce larvae (immature forms). These larvae penetrate the skin, usually of the feet (occasionally producing a rash), and pass through the lungs (producing a cough), to arrive in the small intestine, where they attach themselves by means of teeth or cutting plates. There are two principal species of hookworm which affect man in this way, *Ancylostoma duodenale*, and *Necator americanus*, both of which are small nematodes (roundworms). The worms, which are no longer than about 1cm (½in), continually suck blood from their host at their points of attachment. The main manifestation of hookworm disease, is, not surprisingly, *anaemia*, due to chronic blood loss and iron deficiency. There may be pallor, fatigue, and breathlessness. In severe cases, heart failure and death may occur from this pernicious vampirism.

Obviously, there is much to be said for not walking barefooted in the tropics and subtropics. Both *creeping eruption* and *strongyloidiasis* may be acquired in a similar manner (see *Section 16*).

The most important aspect of therapy is the replacement of iron reserves with *iron supplements*, preferably in combination with foods rich in vitamin C. Where human hookworm is endemic, and reinfection extremely likely, this treatment by itself will usually suffice.

Lymphatic filariasis

Filarial worms are long thread-like roundworms which inhabit the tissues. Lymphatic filariasis, a disease of urban and rural areas of the hot and humid tropics, is caused by *Wuchereria bancrofti* and *Brugia malayi*, both of which are transmitted by mosquitoes. There may be no symptoms after transmission, or there may be recurrent, painful inflammation of the testicles, or the lymph-glands in the arm-pit or groin. In the casual traveller, the disease usually resolves spontaneously, with no permanent disabilities. Serious problems only arise in those residents of endemic areas who are subject to repeated infection. Blockage of the lymphatic system leads to gross and disfiguring swelling of arms, legs, and scrotum (*elephantiasis*).

Homoeopathically, the remedies *Hydrocotyle, Silicea*, or *Anacardium* [*6–30th potency 12h*] have been suggested to moderate the symptoms or course of elephantiasis.

Loiasis (African eye worm/Loa loa)

This filarial worm infection, transmitted by the bite of the large red *Chrysops* fly, is found in the tropical rain-forest and rubber plantation areas of Africa. The fly bites in the day, is associated with forest streams, dislikes open sun, and is attracted by wood-smoke. The initial bite causes a painful swelling, which may persist for 7 days. After an incubation period of several months or longer, there appear the characteristic *Calabar swellings*, lumps some 10cm (4in) or more in diameter. These swellings may appear anywhere on the body, but are more common on the limbs. Their appearance is often preceded by pain or itching, they remain for some hours or days, only to disappear, and recur at a later date. They may do so for up to 18 years. Occasionally, a worm will be seen wriggling across the eye, just under the conjunctiva, this being associated with irritation, pain, and swelling. The worm takes about 30 minutes to traverse the eye, leaving those symptoms in its wake. Fortunately, apart from the annoyance of the condition, serious consequences are rare. Homoeopathically, *Sulphur 6 12h* might be tried.

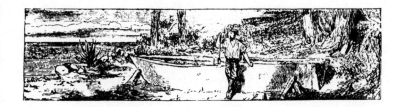

THE HOMOEOPATHIC TRAVEL PACK

Before embarking upon any journey abroad it is wise to equip yourself with at least a basic homoeopathic remedy pack. Obviously, personal requirements will differ greatly, and it is quite possible that you may wish to determine your own by following the guidance of this manual, and the advice of an homoeopathic pharmacist or practitioner. For those who wish for some fundamental direction in this matter, the list of remedies given in this section should be found helpful. To this may then be added any others that would seem appropriate.

For normal purposes, most remedies should be ordered as pilules in 7g vials. Where compactness or weight are important considerations, 1g vials of coarse granules (globules) are preferable. With regard to liquid preparations, including mother tinctures (ø), the minimum quantity to order is 10ml. For creams, the minimum quantity should be 30g (1oz). Glass vials or bottles are desirable, but, where damage is likely to occur, plastic is a better material. For protection against sunlight, such containers should be amber or opaque.

In addition to your selected homoeopathic remedies, you

315

should take with you a good supply of plasters, gauze dressings, ordinary bandages, and crepe bandages. A spare 10ml amber glass dropper-bottle is useful, if you wish to prepare eye-drops (glass is easier to clean for reuse). Those going to exotic places, who may require orthodox treatment, will protect themselves against blood-borne disease by taking with a quantity of presterilized disposable plastic syringes and needles.

INTERNAL REMEDIES (26)

Aconite 30	Hypericum 30
Arnica 30	Ipecacuanha 6
Arsenicum album 6	Ledum 30
Belladonna 30	Mercurius corrosivus 30
Bryonia 30	Nux vomica 30
Cantharis 30	Pulsatilla 6
Carbo vegetabilis 30	Rhus toxicodendron 30
Cinchona officinalis 30	Ruta graveolens 30
Cocculus indicus 30	Silicea 6
Crataegus ø	Sulphur 6
Cuprum metallicum 30	Symphytum 6
Gunpowder 6	Urtica urens ø
Hepar sulphuris 6	Zingiber ø

EXTERNAL REMEDIES (6)

Cremor Calendulae 5% [Calendula cream 5%]
Euphrasia ø
Insect bite application [formula in Section 14]
* Oleum Citronellae [Citronella oil]
* Aqua Rosae Triplex [Triple Rose Water]
Sunburn cream [formula in Section 12]

* Aromatic substances such as these should be packed separately from those bearing a potency number.

INDEX OF PHARMACIES

Some of you will be fortunate enough to have in your area a pharmacy which dispenses homoeopathic remedies. For the remainder, and where difficulty is experienced in obtaining any particular remedy, the following homoeopathic pharmacies offer both an extensive and excellent national and international postal service:

Ainsworths Homoeopathic Pharmacy
38 New Cavendish Street
London W1M 7LH
England
Tel: (071) 935 5330
Fax: (071) 486 4313

Brauer Biotherapies
1 Para Road
PO Box 234
Tanunda
South Australia 5352
Tel: (085) 63 2932
Fax: (085) 63 3398

Standard Homeopathic
210 West 131st Street
Box 61067
Los Angeles
California 90061
USA
Tel: (800) 624 9659
Fax: (213) 516 8579

When dialling from outside the country, please check the international dialling code with your operator.

INDEX

Illnesses and plants have been indexed by both their colloquial and scientific names to enable users to find information quickly.

319

321

Plague, 22–3, 137, 271–3
Plantago major, for scalp ringworm, 189
Plantago major (Greater Plantain), for
    stings, 152
Plantar warts, 210–11
Plumber's itch, 197–8
Plumbum metallicum, for sleeping
    sickness, 304
Plumeria cellinus, for snake bites, 164
Plum stones, 98
Pneumonic plague, 272, 273 *and see*
    plague
Podalgia, 205
Podophyllum for
   diarrhoea, 65
   haemorrhoids, 77
   roundworms, 309
Poison ivy (*Toxicodendron radicans/Rhus
    toxicodendron*), 202
   rash, 201–3
Poison oak (*Toxicodendron
    diversilobum/quercifolium*), 202
Poison sumac (*Toxicodendron vernix*),
    202
Poisonings, 94–109
Polio/Poliomyelitis, 20, 290
Polycarpaea corymbosa, for snake bites,
    165
Polygala senega, for snake bites, 164
Pork tapeworm, 310 *and see* tapeworm
Portuguese man-o'-war (*Physalia
    physalis*), 174
Postural oedema/edema, 31–2
Potato (*Solanum tuberosum*) poisoning,
    102 *and see* poisonings
Potency, 3–4, 6
Powders, 2
Pregnancy, 47–50
Premature ageing, 123–6
Prenanthes serpentaria, for snake bites,
    164
Prescribing, 9–12
Prevention, 13–24
Prickly heat, 121–2 *and see* heat
Prickly pear (*Opuntia spp.*), for stings,
    152
Primary screw worm fly, 196
Protozoan diseases, 134
Prunella vulgaris (Common selfheal), for
    carbuncle, 185
Pseudomonas pseudomallei bacterium,
    279
Psychotria jackii, for snake bites, 165
Pterygium, 230
Ptiloria tenuifolia, for snake bites, 164
Pulex irritans, for insect bites, 146
Pulsatilla for
   breast-feeding, 51, 52
   brucellosis, 276
   caterpillar hair irritation, 200

giardiasis, 68
ill-effects of greasy/fatty foods, 93
malaria, 241–2
measles, 224
mumps, 224
otomycosis, 191
sty, 230
tropical sprue, 72
Pumpkin seeds (*Cucurbita pepo/maxima*),
    for tapeworm, 310
Purple coneflower (*Echinacea
    angustifolia*) for
   snake bites, 164
   stings, 146, 151
Puss caterpillar (*Megalopyge opercularis*),
    200
Pyrethrum, in insect repellent, 140, 141,
    142
Pyrogen for
   animal bites, 181
   pig bel, 103

Q
Q fever and *nosode*, 296 *and see* fevers
Quassia, for lice, 193
Quercus glandium spiritus for
   alcohol craving, 94
   kala azar, 300
   malaria, 244
Quinsy, 222

R
Rabbit fever, 273 *and see* fevers
Rabies, 21–2, 180
Ranunculus bulbosus, for shingles, 226
Ratanhia, for pterygium, 230
Rattlesnakes, 155, 156
Rectal ulcer, 79, 82 *and see* ulcers
Recurrent fever, 273–5 *and see* fevers
Red kidney beans, 109
Red tides, 105
Rehydration fluids, 62–3, 84
Relapsing fever, 135, 137, 273–5 *and see*
    fevers
Renal colic, 119 *and see* colic
Rescue Remedy (Bach) for
   heat exhaustion/prostration, 116
   nervous disorders, 26
   nosebleed, 220
   physical shock, 217–18
   psychological shock, 217
   snake bites, 159, 161
   stings, 153
Retinal detachment, 228 *and see* eye
    problems
Rhaphidophora pertusa, for snake bites,
    165
Rheumatism, 90
Rhinacanthus nasutas, for scalp
    ringworm, 189

Stigmata maidis (Cornsilk), for cystitis, 53
Stinging tree rash, 203
Stings
  bee/wasp/hornet/yellow jacket/ant,
    150–3
  coelenterate, 176
  fish, 176–8
  hymenopterous, 150–3
  nettle, 203
  scorpion, 170–1
  sea urchin, 178–9
  starfish, 178–9
  and see bites
Storage
  herbal preparations, 11
  homoeopathic remedies, 2–3
Strains
  back, 43–4
  eyes, 228
Stramonium for
  malaria, 244
  plague, 272
  typhoid/paratyphoid, 270
Strongyloidiasis, 73, 198, 313
Strontium carbonicum, for ankle/knee
    sprains, 208
Sty(e), 230 *and see* eye problems
Sugar, 8, 93
Sulphur for
  amoebic dysentery, 80–1
  bacillary dysentery, 76
  caterpillar hair irritation, 200
  creeping eruption, 198
  giardiasis, 68
  leprosy, 278
  lice, 193
  loiasis, 314
  mite dermatitis, 147
  onchocerciasis, 234
  scabies, 192
  tropical sprue, 72
Sulphur,
  flowers of, 141
Sun, effects of, 5, 110–26
Surfer's ear, 190–1 *and see* earache
Surgical spirit, for cold sores, 186
Sweating, 111, 114
Sweet fern (*Comptonia peregrina*), for
    poison ivy, 203
Sweet potatoes (*Ipomoea batatas*), 103
Swimmer's cramp, 207
Swimmer's eye, 229–30 *and see* eye
    problems
Swimmer's itch, 198–9 *and see* skin
    problems
Swimming pool earache, 223 *and see*
    earache
Swollen feet, 31–2
Symphytum for
  black eye, 227

fractures, 216
  sprained wrist, 219
  officinale, for solar skin cancer, 126
Syrupus Ficorum, for constipation, 58
Syzygium, for Mexican poppy poisoning,
    100

T
Tabacum, for travel-sickness, 39
Tabernaemontana sralensis, for snake
    bites, 165
Tablets, 2
Tacca fatsiifolia/palmata, for snake bites,
    165
Taenia
  saginata tapeworm, 309
  solium tapeworm 310
Tailbone, bruised, 219
Taipan, 156
Tamus, for chilblains, 131
Tapeworms, 198, 309–12
Tapioca, 96
Tarantulas, 166–7 *and see* spider bites
Tarentula cubensis, for carbuncle, 184
Tartar Emetic (Antimony Potassium
    Tartrate), for bilharziasis, 252
Tea, 109
  for conjunctivitis, 229
  for cystitis, 54
Teak, reactions to, 204
Tellurium for
  body ringworm, 188
  pityriasis versicolor, 190
Temuline, 101
Tennis elbow, 219
Tepeguaje, for casts, 216
Terebinthina for
  bilharziasis, 252
  typhoid/paratyphoid, 271
Tetanus, 20–1
Tetrodotoxic fish poisoning, 104 *and see*
    poisonings
Tetrodotoxin for fish poisoning, 104, 105,
    107
Teucrium marum, for roundworms, 308
Theridion, for nervous disorders, 27
Thiosinaminum, for leishmaniasis, 262
Thirst, 111–12
Threadworms, 306–7
Throats, 222
Thrush, 52–3
Thuja for
  bartonellosis, 277
  bilharziasis, 252
  dermatitis verrucosa, 213
  injection reactions, 16
  leishmaniasis, 264
  prickly heat, 122
  shellfish poisoning, 105
  verrucas, 210

336